EVOLVING CONCEPTS IN SEPSIS AND SEPTIC SHOCK

PERSPECTIVES ON CRITICAL CARE INFECTIOUS DISEASES
Jordi Rello, M.D., Series Editor

---

1. N. Singh and J.M. Aguado (eds.): Infectious Complications in Transplant Recipients. 2000. ISBN 0-7923-7972-1
2. P.Q. Eichacker and J. Pugin (eds.): Evolving Concepts in Sepsis and Septic Shock. 2001. ISBN 0-7923-7235-2

EVOLVING CONCEPTS IN SEPSIS AND SEPTIC SHOCK

Edited by

Peter Q. Eichacker, M.D.
Critical Care Medicine Department
Warren Grant Magnuson Clinical Center
National Institutes of Health
10 Center Drive
Building 10, Room 7D43
Bethesda, MD 20892

and

Jérôme Pugin, M.D.
Division of Medical Intensive Care
University Hospital of Geneva
CH-1211
Geneva 14
Switzerland

KLUWER ACADEMIC PUBLISHERS
Boston/Dordrecht/London

Distributors for North, Central and South America:
Kluwer Academic Publishers
101 Philip Drive
Assinippi Park
Norwell, Massachusetts 02061 USA
Telephone (781) 871-6600
Fax (781) 681-9045
E-Mail <kluwer@wkap.com>

Distributors for all other countries:
Kluwer Academic Publishers Group
Distribution Centre
Post Office Box 322
3300 AH Dordrecht, THE NETHERLANDS
Telephone 31 78 6392 392
Fax 31 78 6392 254
E-Mail <services@wkap.nl>

Electronic Services <http://www.wkap.nl>

Library of Congress Cataloging-in-Publication Data

Evolving concepts in sepsis and septic shock / edited by Peter Q. Eichacker and Jérôme Pugin.
p. ; cm. -- (Perspectives on critical care infectious diseases ; 2)
Includes bibliographical references and index.
ISBN 0-7923-7235-2 (hardback : alk. paper)
1. Septicemia. 2. Septic shock. I. Eichacker, Peter Q. II. Pugin, Jérôme. III. Series.
[DNLM: 1. Sepsis. 2. Anti-Inflammatory Agents--therapeutic use. 3. Shock, Septic.
WC 240 E93 2001]
RC182.S4 E96 2001
616.9'44--dc21

00-048485

Printed on acid-free paper.

Printed in the United States of America

CONTENTS

CONTRIBUTORS

Alain Cariou, M.D.
Medical Intensive Care Unit,
Cochin Port-Royal University Hospital
Paris, France

Thierry Calandra, M.D., Ph.D.
Division of Infectious Diseases
Department of Internal Medicine
Centre Hospitalier Universitaire Vaudois
Lausanne, Switzerland

R. Phillip Dellinger, M.D.
Rush-Presbyterian-St. Luke's Medical Center
Chicago, Illinois

Jean-François Dhainaut, M.D., Ph.D.
Medical Intensive Care Unit
Cochin Port-Royal University Hospital
Paris, France

Wolf-Dietrich Döcke, M.D.
Institute of Medical Immunology and
Department of Nephrology and Internal Intensive Medicine
Humboldt-University Berlin
Berlin, Germany

Peter Q. Eichacker, M.D.
Critical Care Medicine Department
Clinical Center
National Institutes of Health,
Bethesda, MD

Bradley D. Freeman, M.D.
Departments of Surgery
Washington University School of Medicine
St. Louis, MO

Sergey Goodman, M.D., Ph.D.
Hadassah Hebrew University Medical Center
Department of Anesthesiology and Critical Care Medicine
Jerusalem, Israel

Nathalie Marin, Ph.D.
Medical Intensive Care Unit
Cochin Port-Royal University Hospital
Paris, France

Christian Martin, Ph.D.
Division of Infectious Diseases
Department of Internal Medicine
Centre Hospitalier Universitaire Vaudois
Lausanne, Switzerland

G. Umberto Meduri, M.D.
Memphis Lung Research Program, Department of Medicine Divisions of Pulmonary and Critical Care Medicine and Infectious Disease and Department of Preventive Medicine
University of Tennessee, Memphis and Veterans Affairs Medical Center
Memphis, Tennessee

Charles Natanson, M.D.
Critical Care Medicine Department
Clinical Center National Institutes of Health
Bethesda, MD

Chantal Parent, D.V.M.
Critical Care Medicine Department
Clinical Center
National Institutes of Health
Bethesda, MD

Javier Pérez, M.D.
Rush-Presbyterian-St. Luke's Medical Center
Chicago, Illinois

Jérôme Pugin, M.D.
Division of Medical Intensive Care
University Hospital of Geneva
Geneva, Switzerland

Petra Reinke, M.D., Ph.D.
Institute of Medical Immunology and
Department of Nephrology and Internal Intensive Medicine
Humboldt-University Berlin
Berlin, Germany

Thierry Roger, Ph.D.
Division of Infectious Diseases
Department of Internal Medicine
Centre Hospitalier Universitaire Vaudois
Lausanne, Switzerland

Robert Sabat, M.D.
Institute of Medical Immunology and
Department of Nephrology and Internal Intensive Medicine
Humboldt-University Berlin
Berlin, Germany

Jonathan Sevransky, M.D.
Johns Hopkins University School of Medicine
Division of Pulmonary and Critical Care Medicine
Baltimore, MD

Charles L. Sprung, M.D.
Hadassah Hebrew University Medical Center
Department of Anesthesiology and Critical Care Medicine
Jerusalem, Israel

Frank Stüber, M.D.
University of Bonn
Department of Anesthesiology and Intensive Care Medicine
Bonn, Germany

Jean-Louis Vincent, M.D.
Erasme Hospital
Department of Intensive Care
Free University of Brussels
Brussels, Belgium

Hans-Dieter Volk, M.D., Ph.D.
Institute of Medical Immunology and Department of Nephrology and Internal Intensive Medicine
Humboldt-University Berlin
Berlin, Germany

Kerstin Wolk, Ph.D
Institute of Medical Immunology and Department of Nephrology and Internal Intensive Medicine,
Humboldt-University Berlin
Berlin, Germany

Barbara A. Zehnbauer, Ph.D.
Department of Pathology
Washington University School of Medicine
St. Louis, MO

Preface

Much research over the past 30 to 40 years has shown that the inflammatory response, while critical for host defense during microbial infection, may itself play a central role in the pathogenesis of sepsis. Although key mediators responsible for this injury have been identified, efforts clinically to augment our conventional antimicrobial and supportive therapies during sepsis with agents modulating the inflammatory response have been unsuccessful. As a result, the mortality associated with this lethal syndrome, especially when complicated by shock, has remained persistently high. Unfortunately, during this same period of time, the incidence of sepsis has accelerated as other fields of medicine have relied increasingly on therapies which predispose to infection.

While frustrating, overall this experience in the field of sepsis has not been without value. Most importantly, it has helped define on several different levels the complexity of the septic patient. Recognizing and addressing this complexity as discussed by each of the contributors to this volume may now be providing new inroads into the treatment of sepsis.

One of the greatest problems researchers have faced is accurately and uniformly defining a target population of patients. Both the nonspecificity of elements in the host inflammatory response as well as the often obscure nature of the infectious focus frequently makes identification of the patient with sepsis difficult. The chapters by Dr's Perez and Dellinger and by Dr Vincent both highlight the importance of this problem as well as provide insights into ways to address it. Although much is now known about the host inflammatory response in sepsis, this is an extremely complex reaction about which much more still needs to be learned. Critical new components in our evolving picture of this response are presented in chapters by Dr. Pugin and

Drs. Martin, Roger and Calandra. Furthermore, as discussed by Dr's Freeman and Zehnbauer and by Dr. Stüber, there is now accumulating data to indicate that an individual's genetic background may contribute importantly to the quality and intensity of this inflammatory response.

To date several different types of antiinflammatory therapies of been tested in patients with sepsis. Our early experience was with high dose cortiocosteroids, a nonspecific type of agent which ultimately was shown not to be beneficial in large controlled trials. In the chapters by Dr's Goodman and Sprung and by Dr. Meduri, this prior experience is described while newer findings supporting a very different approach for the use of corticosteroids in sepsis are presented. Our more recent experience with mediator-specific antiinflammatory agents in sepsis will be discussed in chapters by Dr's Sevransky and Natanson and by Drs. Dhainaut, Marin, and Cariou. Although these agents have also been disappointing in clinical trials, overall results from these studies do provide evidence that inhibiting the inflammatory response in sepsis will be beneficial in some patients, thus supporting further work with this therapeutic approach. Finally, while limiting an excessive inflammatory response has been a prominent goal in the treatment of sepsis, emerging data suggests that in some patients, an inadequate response and poor host defense may be a greater problem. In such patients, augmenting this response with proinflammatory agents may in fact be beneficial. The chapters by Drs. Eichacker, Parent, Volk, Wolk, Sabat, Docke, Reinke and by Drs. Parent and Eichacker discuss this different therapeutic approach.

Overall, this volume should provide the reader with insights into some of the most interesting and potentially useful new developments in the field of sepsis. We are very grateful to each of the contributors for the time and effort they have expended to make this an exciting and useful reference. We also wish to thank Dr. Jordi Rello for giving us the opportunity to prepare this volume in his Perspectives Series. Finally, we are very thankful to Ms. Jennifer Candotti for her exceptional editorial assistance during its preparation.

Peter Q. Eichacker MD
Jérôme Pugin MD
Guest Editors

Chapter 1

SEPSIS DEFINITIONS

Javier Pérez, M.D., R. Phillip Dellinger, M.D.
Rush-Presbyterian-St. Luke's Medical Center Chicago, Illinois

What is sepsis?

Stedman's medical dictionary defines sepsis as "the presence of various pus-forming and other pathogenic organisms, or their toxins, in the blood or tissues" (1).

Sepsis has been a term used since ancient times to describe severe or life-threatening infections. In the past, the presence of systemic manifestations, including organ dysfunction remote from the site of infection, and a recognized site of infection were typically required to define sepsis (2,3).

In the last three decades, sepsis has become a more prominent reason for ICU admission and hospital death. Supportive medical care has improved and we now have the ability to prolong life in disease states, which before had little hope for longevity. Likewise, acute life-threatening conditions, previously associated with an ominous prognosis, are now associated with longer survival rates and prolonged stays in critical care units. This increase in survival in critically ill patients is in turn associated with a higher risk of life-threatening infection. In addition, it is now recognized that severe insults other than infection can produce a generalized systemic reaction and multi-organ dysfunction indistinguishable from those induced by sepsis.

Many authors question the requirement for the presence of a documented infection to define sepsis (4-6). There are patients who, having systemic manifestations of infection, do not have evidence of infection. There are similar patients who, although having a clear clinical source of infection, have no organisms isolated from the source.

The need for standard definition

Throughout the first two thirds of the twentieth-century, authors and practicing physicians used multiple terms to define patients with serious manifestations of infection. Commonly used to confer more serious prognosis to the infection, terms like sepsis, bacteremia, septicemia and septic shock were interchanged in the medical literature to describe the same patients. The appearance of large clinical trials in the mid-eighties testing the efficacy of innovative anti-inflammatory therapies is the origin of a great part of the debate on sepsis definitions. Different characterizations of sepsis, using terms such as septicemia and septic shock, were used for enrollment into clinical trials making comparison of results difficult or impossible. A new term, sepsis syndrome, appeared to describe patients with clinical evidence of infection and some pre-defined combination of systemic manifestations of infection (i.e. temperature changes, tachycardia, tachypnea and an evidence of organ dysfunction or hypotension) (7-8). Motivated by the occurrence of sepsis in almost half a million Americans every year (9) and considering the need to standardize terminology used for enrollment in clinical trials, two scientific organizations in the U.S. sponsored a consensus conference in hope of providing standard terminology for sepsis definitions (10). The consensus conference was also motivated by the desire of industry to insure that criteria used in large expensive sepsis trials would meet approval of the academic community. The definitions established in the consensus conference and the response of the scientific community to those definitions will be extensively discussed in this manuscript.

Knowledge of the epidemiology of sepsis and its sequelae is increasingly important. As new treatment modalities, every day more expensive, are being subjected to clinical trials, our need for better definitions that accurately reflect new pathophysiologic pathways, mediators and markers, becomes an urgent necessity.

SEPSIS IN THE MEDICAL LITERATURE

Before the consensus

Two decades ago, the link between infection and systemic abnormalities of body function was solidified and the idea of microbial induced "sepsis" was established. Bacteremia was required by some investigators to define sepsis for the purpose of clinical trials. The term *bacteremia* was even used as entrance criteria in a large multicenter trial (7). The relation between the presence of sepsis associated with gram-negative bacteremia, and antibiotic effect on survival was also demonstrated (2). Gram-negative bacteremia was seen synonymously as sepsis in this study.

The importance of the organism's response to an infectious insult was soon recognized as an equal and sometimes greater determinant of outcome. This inflammatory response was defined as the *sepsis syndrome* (7). Moreover, the presence of a similar inflammatory reaction in patients affected by non-infectious conditions such as pancreatitis and burns was also recognized (5). The role of the inflammatory response as it affects the survival of septic patients was widely discussed (14). The pathophysiology of the infection became better understood. The association between interleukin-1 and fever (15) and the role of tumor necrosis factor in the host-derived reaction (16) changed our knowledge of the inflammatory response of the body against infection. Other products were also implicated in this inflammatory reaction such as interleukin-2, interleukin-6, interleukin-8 and prostaglandin E2, together with the important roles of oxygen free radicals and the coagulation pathways. Similar inflammatory reactions were seen with non-infectious insults (5, 17). It was thought that patients who died early with sepsis-induced cardiovascular dysfunction, versus those who died later due to sepsis-induced organ failure, likely had an overwhelming cytokine response that was driving early deaths. Clinical trials confirmed that patients with shock and increased number of organ dysfunctions had decreased survival (7). The development of organ failure as a cause of later deaths was also thought to be related to cytokine effects. Large clinical trials were designed in hopes of demonstrating that antiinflammatory therapy could control this inflammatory response and improve survival (18-22).

Although clinical trials failed to demonstrate any beneficial effect of new therapies, a remarkable variety in mortality rates of patients with sepsis, sepsis syndrome and septic shock was noted. Mortality associated with septic shock was reported to range from 10 to 90% (23). Many reasons were suggested to explain this disparity, but the variation in how sepsis and septic shock was defined from study to study was largely thought to be responsible for this difference (24-25). This definition problem existed not only with terms used for entrance into clinical trials but also for classifications of subgroups within the trial.

It was difficult to compare sepsis study results when different definitions were used for the same term. The medical literature in sepsis was described as a "tower of Babel" (26), in which each author applied his/her own significance for definitions of sepsis.

THE CONSENSUS CONFERENCE

In August 1991, a group of experienced clinicians involved in sepsis research gathered in Chicago in an attempt to provide some order and standardization to the sepsis definitions (10). With the proliferation of new innovative therapeutic agents entering clinical trials in sepsis, more precise and standardized definitions were needed to allow comparison of trials and more relevant definitions were needed to use as entrance criteria to optimize chances for a successful study.

Months earlier, Roger C. Bone had published two additional articles (25, 27) in an attempt to establish uniform criteria for sepsis definitions. Two articles replying to those definitions questioned Dr. Bone's definition proposal (5,8). Controversy centered on the use of the term sepsis in non-infectious conditions and how should non-infectious but sepsis-like conditions be defined. The need for precise nomenclature describing infection induced organ dysfunction and failure, the usefulness of the terms septicemia and sepsis syndrome, a precise definition of septic shock, what level of systemic abnormality would be linked to the term "sepsis", and establishing gradations of sepsis, if any, were the fundamental issues addressed at the 1991 Consensus Conference.

The Consensus Conference agreed on definitions for the term bacteremia, sepsis, severe sepsis and septic shock. The definitions established by the consensus conference are summarized in Table 1.

A singular proposal of the consensus conference was to recognize sepsis and its sequelae as a continuum. The systemic response could manifest before signs of the infection and alert the physician to search for infections, and sepsis may be premonitory of severe sepsis and septic shock. It was hoped that the early diagnosis and treatment of sepsis might minimize the impact of these later events and limit the development of organ dysfunction. When an organ dysfunction secondary to sepsis occurs, it was defined with the term *severe sepsis*. When hypotension occurs, and was non-responsive to fluids, requiring vasopressor support and associated with hypoperfusion abnormalities, it was defined as *septic shock*.

Certainly, the most original contribution of the consensus conference was the creation of the term SIRS, to express *systemic inflammatory response syndrome*. The term was coined to describe evidence of systemic inflammation due to an infectious or non-infectious process. SIRS could be due to infection or non-infectious insults such as pancreatitis, burns and multi-systemic trauma. The threshold for SIRS required achieving at least two out of four criteria (see Table 1). Only when SIRS is associated with infection is it defined as sepsis.

Table 1. Summary of the consensus conference definitions

Infection: Microbial phenomenon characterized by an inflammatory response to the presence of microorganisms or the invasion of normally sterile host tissue by those organisms.

Bacteremia: The presence of viable bacteria in the blood.

Systemic Inflammatory Response Syndrome (SIRS): The systemic inflammatory response to a variety of severe clinical insults. The response is manifested by two or more of the following conditions:

Temperature > 38° or < 36° C
Heart rate > 90 beats/min
Respiratory rate > 20 breaths/min or $PaCO_2$ < 32 torr (<4.3 kPa)
WBC > 12,000 cells/mm^3, <4000 cells/ mm^3, or > 10% immature (band) forms

Sepsis: The systemic response to infection. This systemic response is manifested by two or more of the above conditions (SIRS) as a result of infection.

Severe sepsis: Sepsis associated with organ dysfunction, hypoperfusion or hypotension. Hypoperfusion and perfusion abnormalities may include, but are not limited to, lactic acidosis, oliguria or acute alteration of mental status.

Sepsis Shock: Sepsis with hypotension, despite adequate fluid resuscitation, along with the presence of perfusion abnormalities that may include, but are not limited to, lactic acidosis, oliguria or acute alteration in mental status. Patients who are on inotropic or vasopressor agents may not be hypotensive at the time that perfusion abnormalities are measured

Sepsis induced hypotension: a systolic BP of < 90 mm Hg or a reduction of > 40 mm Hg from baseline in the absence of other causes for hypotension

Multiple Organ Dysfunction Syndrome: Presence of altered organ function in an acutely ill patient such that homeostasis cannot be maintained without intervention

The Consensus Conference linked sepsis to infection and iterated that the term should not be used in the absence of a clinical diagnosis (i.e., subcutaneous abscess). Ideally the term would apply when a bacteriologically confirmed diagnosis of infection (i.e., bacteremia, confirmed gram stain or culture from the abscess) was present.

The second major decision related to the definition of sepsis was that it was assigned to be present beginning at a low level of SIRS manifestations (merely the presence of SIRS and a documented infection). At the time of the consensus conference some used the term sepsis to define a previously healthy female with pyelonephritis and high temperature and leukocytosis, while others used the term to describe a patient admitted to the ICU with infection-induced hypotension and organ dysfunction. A decision had to be made to either use the former, the latter, or neither as a threshold for sepsis. Since SIRS had been established as the threshold for insult-induced inflammation, the decision was made to determine sepsis as the lowest level of infection-induced systemic inflammation. A new term, "severe sepsis" was then created to describe the patient with life-threatening sepsis and included evidence of sepsis-induced organ dysfunction, hypoperfusion abnormality or hypotension.

Sepsis-induced hypotension and septic shock were given very specific definitions, and types of hypoperfusion abnormalities were elucidated. Since there was no literature guidance to allow identification of thresholds for organ dysfunction (liver, kidney, coagulation), these thresholds were not established.

Finally two terms that meant many different things to many different people were recommended to be abandoned: *sepsis syndrome* (which previously signified the presence of infection for some and a sepsis-like condition for others) and *septicemia* (which meant sepsis and bacteremia to some and severe systemic infectious manifestations of infection to others).

The definitions established in the consensus conference were based on physiologic variables. The members of the consensus conference recognized a lack in our knowledge base of sepsis. An understanding of the incidence, natural history and outcome of sepsis was poorly developed at that time. For those reasons, the definitions established in the consensus conference have subsequently drawn criticism (6, 11-13). Most of these critiques present valid points, most prominently that the definitions are based on physiologic variables and do not contemplate the pathophysiologic mechanisms, biological markers or temporal sequence of sepsis and its etiology. Defining sepsis as a single disease, or implying that all patients who develop sepsis share the same pathophysiologic mechanisms is something that we know today is incorrect. Finally, the consensus conference defined sepsis as a continuum, with the most feared sequelae of sepsis being severe sepsis, septic shock and multiple organ dysfunction. However, the consensus never defined a similar progression for SIRS and evidence of non-infectious-induced organ dysfunction.

The members of the consensus conference recognized the limitations in the definitions and pleaded for research that would allow better definitions of sepsis and its mechanisms in the future.

SEPSIS: CLINICAL SIGNIFICANCE

SIRS: The controversy

Introduced to define patients who developed systemic inflammatory reaction against both infectious and non-infectious insults, the term SIRS had its detractors from the very beginning (8). SIRS was "accused" of being too sensitive, too non-specific and even of being dangerous since it reduced the physician's incentive in searching for infectious sources in patients with SIRS and no obvious source of infection (12).

However, the idea of SIRS, and how it was intended to be used, was defended by others (26, 28). With sepsis defined as a continuum, SIRS and infection was defined as a low threshold for sepsis. In 1995, Rangel-Frausto et al. (29) published the first prospective study attempting to define the natural history of SIRS. The authors concluded that the presence of three or more criteria of SIRS (Table 1) was helpful to define a subgroup of patients, either on the ICU or on the ward, who were at special risk of development sepsis. In that study the hypothesis of SIRS representing the lowest in the hierarchy of SIRS→sepsis→severe sepsis→septic shock was also proven.

The definition of the term SIRS was also important as it helped to separate those insults that create systemic inflammatory reactions but that are not related to infection. It has been observed that SIRS can progress to organ dysfunction either in the absence of infection (pancreatitis) or when infection is suspected but the source cannot be identified. Large clinical trials in severe infection used the term SIRS and the criteria defined in SIRS for patients to be included in those trials (30, 31). Some studies demonstrated the relation between the presence of SIRS and further development of more severe states such as multiple organ dysfunction (29, 32). Others, however, accused the term SIRS of being useless to predict severity of disease (6, 33).

A common complaint is that the definition of SIRS does not contemplate the existence of a continuum of the development of multiple organ dysfunction from SIRS in the absence of infection. For that reason, some authors have advocated the creation of the term severe SIRS to imply development of organ dysfunction, hypoperfusion abnormalities or hypotension in the absence of clinical evidence of infection (32, 34).

Sepsis and severe sepsis in clinical trials

Overall, more than 12,500 patients have been enrolled in clinical trials of sepsis. The heterogeneity of these patients is thought to be problematic (13). Trials using anti-inflammatory drugs have included septic patients with urinary tract infection and those with aspiration pneumonia under the same umbrella. It is unlikely that the clinical prognosis of these two patient groups is the same. Despite attempts to tighten the criteria for enrollment in clinical trials of severe sepsis, the variability in some studies remains bothersome. Chronic health conditions also play a major role in the prognosis of septic patients. Obviously none of these factors are covered in the consensus definitions. In addition, the pathophysiology included in the consensus definitions does not represent a precise biologic inflammatory profile. It is this profile that is likely the most important predictor of success or failure of immunologic therapy.

The consensus conference's definitions did not intend to predict outcome. However, some clinical studies support that levels of severity and mortality can correlate with the magnitude of the SIRS response. Rangel-Frausto et al. (29) described that almost half of the patients who developed sepsis, severe sepsis or septic shock previously had SIRS, sepsis, or severe sepis respectively. Muckart et al (32) performed a prospective cohort analysis in 450 trauma patients. The authors concluded that the current definitions of SIRS, sepsis and septic shock showed a significant association with physiologic deterioration and increasing organ dysfunction. However, only septic shock had significant influence on mortality.

Unfortunately, despite the consensus conference, inclusion criteria on large sepsis studies performed after the conference were not homogenous. A term that was suggested to be abandoned, sepsis syndrome, continued to be used in large clinical trials of anti-inflammatory drugs (36-39). The term was also used in a multicenter trial in sepsis epidemiology (35). In that study, the authors concluded that there was a continuum in the development of septic shock from earlier states, although they used the term sepsis syndrome to define those previous states. They also concluded that the terms SIRS and sepsis describe a significant proportion of patients with low risk of developing further morbid conditions.

Many critiques have risen of the consensus conference sepsis definitions. The definitions have been accused of being too sensitive. Two recent studies have documented that more than 90% of the ICU admission met SIRS criteria, without necessarily developing sepsis, severe sepsis, septic shock or multiple organ dysfunction (6, 32). The definitions have also been accused of being non-specific, allowing a wide variety of patients with different pathology to be included in the clinical trials.

Multiple clinical trials have been conducted to research specific anti-inflammatory therapies in sepsis. Subgroup analysis of the placebo arm of these studies suggests that a more rigorous definition that included biological profiles could lead to a benefit in certain group of patients. For example, in the study by Martin et al (40), a relation between the levels of TNF-alpha concentration and survival from septic shock was found. Moreover, there was a difference in the levels of Interleukin-6 in septic shock patients when compared with trauma patients, being lower in the second group. Reinhart et al., in a multicenter placebo-controlled trial (44), demonstrated in a subgroup analysis that those patients with high levels of interleukin-6 were more prone to respond to anti-TNF-alpha. Similarly, Abraham et al. (54), in a placebo-controlled trial, suggested that a pre-treatment subgroup analysis could determine better results, as they observed that after applying logistic regression analysis by means of predicted mortality and serum interleukin-6 levels, there was an improvement of patients treated with p55-IgG, the tested substance.

The overall results of clinical trials in the last decade have not been encouraging. Mortality of patients with septic shock continues to vary from 36-60% in these trials, although similar inclusion criteria and populations were used. Based on these results, and since the definitions were used in some of those trials, the utility of the consensus definitions has been widely questioned. Whether a revision of the definitions or newer ones that include biologic and genetic markers will help us to develop better clinical trials is still unresolved.

FUTURE DIRECTIONS

Why has the standardization of definitions not improved our capability to carry out successful trials of innovative immunologic therapy in severe sepsis? Two reasons are clearly identified.

First is our realization that success of immunotherapy is likely equally dependent on the timing of therapy, the activity of the drug and the use of a single agent in such a complex biologic environment.

The second, and perhaps the one that can be ultimately easier to solve is that any clinical classification of patients with sepsis does not reliably predict mediator milieu which would seem to be most important for any therapeutic effect of immunologic therapy. Therefore, the search for mediator profiles that predict response to immunologic therapy is paramount.

Clinical profiles are unlikely to correlate well with underlying biologic profiles. The identification of patients who are likely to benefit from specific immuno-modulation based purely on clinical information is unlikely. For example, it would be inappropriate to initiate insulin therapy for polyuria and polydipsia without knowing serum glucose values. Likewise, it would be inappropriate to consider a patient with chest pain, shortness of breath and diaphoresis as a candidate for thrombolytic therapy based on those clinical signs and the assumption that the patient is suffering an acute myocardial infarction. For the same reason, it is unlikely that white blood cell count, body temperature and even organ injury are specific enough to warrant classification of patients under the same subgroups for the purpose of anti-inflammatory therapy. Moreover, having the same type of insult (e.g. urinary tract infection with *E. coli)* does not preclude having different severities of illness (e.g. sepsis or septic shock). What is likely needed is a biologic profile consisting of a composite picture of pro-inflammatory and anti-inflammatory mediators. The need to ascertain the overall effect of the biologic profile by measuring status of the target cell (turned on-turned off), is also likely needed. Even the genetic regulation for that response may be important in predicting reaction to immunologic therapy.

In recent years we have made considerable progress in the laboratory in unraveling the biologic milieu of sepsis and the complexity of the multiple mediators and feedback pathways. Extensive animal and human studies have focused on the inflammatory reaction secondary to diverse insults (13, 28). Based on these findings we have learned that differences in the initial insult can result in activation of different inflammatory mechanisms (13, 23, 41). We have also learned that coexistent diseases not only predict outcome but also likelihood of development of severe inflammatory reactions (e.g. diabetics have less development of ARDS) (42). We have learned that success of anti-inflammatory therapy may be linked to the etiology of the insult. For example, when gram-positive organisms are the origin of septic shock the response to anti-TNF therapy may be impaired (43).

There is intense interest in establishing relationships among biologic markers of sepsis and stages of sepsis. Elevations of IL-1, IL-6, IL-8, IL-10, TNF-alpha and TNF soluble receptor have been demonstrated in sepsis (44-46). Profiles of these pro-inflammatory and anti-inflammatory mediators are likely to have clinical pertinence (47). Cytokines, interleukins for example, can also be present in high levels in other conditions such as burns, trauma, surgery, chronic liver disease and pancreatitis (48-52).

Promising results were initially obtained in studies of inhibition of TNF-alpha in sepsis. One open-label study with anti-TNF therapy suggested an increase in oxygenation and ventricular function in patients with septic shock (53). Some trials of anti-TNF therapy have measured basal levels of TNF at the time of enrollment (44, 54). Since rapid turn-around assays for TNF are not available, the levels could not be used as a criteria for inclusion. Although no subgroup analysis of patients with elevated TNF levels at the time of enrollment have suggested this group would be more likely to benefit from anti-TNF therapy, other more sophisticated assays of inflammatory profile and status of cellular activation might be more useful (47).

In recent trials, C-reactive protein (CRP) and procalcitonin (PCT) have been used as markers of sepsis (54-56). High levels of CRP have been shown to differentiate bacterial infections from viral infections (57). Decreasing CRP levels predict the recovery phase of sepsis (58-59). Although reported more sensitive than fever or leukocytosis in identifying sepsis, high levels of CRP have also been documented in trauma and surgery, especially cardiac surgery. Ugarte et al (60) found that the combination of CRP and PCT was very specific for infection. However in that study CRP demonstrated greater sensitivity and specificity than PCT for infection. PCT has been demonstrated to be a good marker of infection in patients with pancreatitis (61) and renal transplant (62). Both PCT and CRP are not 100% sensitive or specific. Normal values are probably most useful in defining that infection is unlikely. The ability of these markers to facilitate identification and classification of sepsis is not clear.

CONCLUSIONS

In conclusion, we feel that sepsis definitions are essential to standardize our discussions of sepsis and for the comparison of clinical trial designs. The current definitions are better than none but fall short of predicting response to immunologic therapy, assuming that some patients will benefit from immunologic therapy.

The development of bedside tests to rapidly detect endotoxin and cytokines is an attractive tool that will allow the testing of the hypothesis that biologic profiles may be more useful than clinical definitions based on vital signs, white blood cell count and tests of organ injury and dysfunction in defining presence of sepsis, stage of sepsis and its response to immunologic therapy. The ability to sample endotoxin and cytokines in body compartments and to ascertain cellular status (i.e., turned on or turned off) may be important.

Hopefully, as we continue to refine relationships of biologic profiles to organ injury, we will move closer to the elusive goal of successful immunologic therapy of sepsis.

REFERENCES

1. Stedman's Medical Dictionary. 26th edition. Williams and Wilkins. Baltimore 1995.
2. Kreger BE, Craven DE, McCabe WR. Gram-negative bacteremia. Reevaluation of clinical features and treatment in 612 patients. Am J Med 1980;68: 344-55.
3. Ziegler EJ, McCutchan JA, Fierer J, Glauser MP, Sadoff JC, Douglas H, Braude AI. Treatment of gram-negative bacteremia and shock with human antiserum to a mutant Escherichia coli. N Eng J Med 1982;307: 1225-30.

4. Poole GV, Griswald JA, Mukkassa FF. Sepsis and infection in the intensive care unit: are they related? Am Surg 1993;59: 60-4.
5. Sibbald WJ, Marshall J, Christou N and the Canadian Multiple Organ Failure Study Group. "Sepsis": clarity of existing terminology... or more confusion? Crit Care Med 1991;19: 996-8.
6. Bossink AWJ, Groeneveld J, Hack EC, Thijs LG. Predictor of mortality in febrile medical patients. How useful are "SIRS" and sepsis criteria? Chest 1998;113: 1533-41.
7. Bone RC, Fisher CJ, Clemmer TP, Slotman GJ, Metz CA, Balk RA. Sepsis syndrome: a valid clinical entity. Methylprednisolone Severe Sepsis Study Group. Crit Care Med 1989;17: 389-93.
8. Sprung CL. Definitions of sepsis-Have we reached a consensus? Crit Care Med 1991;19:849-51.
9. Parker MM, Parrillo JE. Septic shock: hemodynamics and pathogenesis. JAMA 1983;250:3324-7.
10. Members of the American College of Chest Physicians/Society of Critical Care Medicine Consensus Conference Committee. Definitions for sepsis and organ failure and guidelines for the use of innovative therapies in sepsis. Crit Care Med 1992;20:864-74.
11. Knaus WA, Sun X, Nystrom O, Wagner DP. Evaluation of definitions for sepsis. Chest 1992;101: 1656-62.
12. Vincent J-L. Dear SIRS, I'm sorry to say that I don't like you... Crit Care Med 1997;25:372-4.
13. Abraham E, Matthay MA, Dinarello CA, Vincent JL, Cohen J, Opal S, Glauser M, Parsons P, Fisher CJ Jr., Repine JE. Consensus conference definitions for sepsis, septic shock, acute lung injury and acute respiratory distress syndrome: Time for a reevaluation. Crit Care Med 2000;28:232-5.
14. Marshall JC, Sweeney D. Microbial infections and the septic response in critical surgical illness. Sepsis, not infection, determines outcome. Arch Surg 1990;125:17-23.
15. Dinarello CA. Interleukin-1 and the pathogenesis of the acute phase response. N Eng J Med 1984;311:1413-8.
16. Beutler B, Cerami A. Cachectin: more than a tumor necrosis factor. N Eng J Med 1987;316:379-85.
17. Watters JM, Bessey PQ, Dinarello CA, Wolff SM, Wilmore DW. Both inflammatory and endocrine mediators stimulate host response to sepsis. Arch Surg 1986;121:179-90
18. Schumer W. Steroids in the treatment of clinical septic shock. Ann Surg 1976;184:333-41.
19. Luce JM, Montgomery AB, Marks JD, Turner J, Metz CA, Murray JF. Ineffectiveness of high dose methyl-prednisolone in preventing parenchymal lung injury and improving mortality in septic shock. Am Rev Respir Dis 1988;138:62-8.
20. The Veterans administration Systemic Sepsis Cooperative Study Group. Effect of high-dose glucocorticoid therapy on mortality in patients with clinical signs of sepsis. N Eng J Med 1987;317:659-65.
21. Bone RC, Fisher CJ, Clemmer TP. A controlled trial of high-dose methylprednisolone in the treatment of severe sepsis and septic shock. N Eng J Med 1987;317:653-8.
22. Sprung CL, Caralis PV, Marcial EG. The effects of high-dose corticosteroids in patients with septic shock: A prospective, controlled study. N Eng J Med 1984;311:1137-43.

23. Zeni F, Freeman B, Natanson C. Anti-inflammatory therapies to treat sepsis and septic shock: A reassessment. Crit Care Med 1997;25:1095-100.
24. Bone RC, Sibbald WJ, Sprung CL. The ACCP-SCCM consensus conference on sepsis and organ failure. Chest 1992;101:1481-3.
25. Bone RC. Let's agree on terminology: definitions of sepsis. Crit Care Med 1991;19:973-6.
26. Dellinger RP, Bone RC. To SIRS with love. Crit Care Med 1998;26:178-179.
27. Bone RC. Sepsis, sepsis syndrome, multi-organ failure: a plea for comparable definitions. Ann Intern Med 1991;114:332-3.
28. Bone RC, Grodzin CJ, Balk RA. Sepsis: a new hypothesis for pathogenesis of the disease process. Chest 1997;112:235-43.
29. Rangel-Frausto MS, Pittet D, Costigan M, Hwang T, Davis CS, Wenzel RP. The natural history of the systemic inflammatory response syndrome (SIRS). JAMA 1995;273:117-23.
30. Forceville X, Vitoux D, Gauzit R, Combes A, Lahilaire P, Chappuis P. Selenium, systemic immune response syndrome, sepsis and outcome in critically ill patients. Crit Care Med 1998;26:1536-44.
31. Fein AM, Bernard GR, Criner GJ, Fletcher EC, Good JT Jr., Knaus WA, Levy H, Matuschak GM, Shanies HM, Taylor RW. Treatment of severe inflammatory response syndrome and sepsis with a novel bradykinin antagonist, Deltibant (CP-0127). JAMA 1997;277:482-7.
32. Muckart DJJ, Bhagwanjee S. American College of Physicians/Society of Critical Care Medicine consensus conference definitions of the systemic inflammatory response syndrome and allied disorders in relation to critically injured patients. Crit Care Med 1997;25:1789-95.
33. Pittet D, Rangel-Frausto S, Li N, Tarara D, Costigan M, Rempe L, Jebson P, Wenzel RP. Systemic inflammatory response syndrome, sepsis, severe sepsis and septic shock: incidence, morbidities and outcomes in surgical ICU patients. Int Care Med 1995;21:302-9.
34. Bernard GR. Sepsis trials: intersection of investigation, regulation, funding and practice. Am J Respir Crit Care Med 1995;152:4-10.
35. Sands KE, Bates DW, Lanken PA, Graman PS, Hibberd PL, Kahn KL, Parsonnet J, Panzer R, Oray EJ, Snydman DR. Epidemiology of sepsis syndrome in 8 academic medical centers. JAMA 1997;278:234-40.
36. Dhainaut JF, Tenaillon A, Le Tulzo Y, Schlemmer B, Solet JP, Wolff M, Holzapfel L, Zeni F, Dreyfuss D, Mira JP. Platelet –activating factor receptor antagonist BN 52021 in the treatment of severe sepsis: a randomized, double-blind, placebo-controlled, multicenter clinical trial. Crit Care Med 1994;22:1720-28.
37. Fisher CJ, Slotman GJ, Opal SM, Pribble JP, Bone RC, Emmanuel G NgD, Bloedow DC, Catalano MA. Initial evaluation of human recombinant interleukin-1 receptor antagonist in the treatment of sepsis syndrome: a randomized, open-label, placebo-controlled multicenter trial. Crit Care Med 1994;22:12-21.
38. Fisher CJ, Dhainaut JF, Opal SM, Pribble JP, Balk RA, Slotman GJ, Iberti TJ, Rackow EC, Shapiro MJ, Greenman RL, Reines D, Shelly MP, Thompson BW, LaBrecque JF, Catalano MA, Knaus WA, Sadoff JC. Recombinant human interleukins-1 receptor antagonist in the treatment of patients with sepsis syndrome. JAMA 1994;271:1836-43.
39. Abraham E, Wunderink R, Silverman H, Perl TM, Nasraway S, Levy H, Bone R, Wenzel RP, Balk R, Allred R, Pennington JE, Wherry JC. Efficacy and safety of

monoclonal antibody to human tumor necrosis factor alpha inpatients with sepsis syndrome: a randomized, controlled, double-blind, multicenter trial. JAMA 1995;273:934-41.

40. Martin C, Boisson C, Haccoun M, Thomachot L, Mege JL. Patterns of cytokine evolution, tumor necrosis factor-alpha and interleukin-6 after septic shock, hemorrhagic shock and severe trauma. Crit Care Med 1997;25:1813-19.
41. Folkesson HG, Matthay MA, Hebert CA, Broaddus VC. Acid aspiration-induced lung injury in rabbits is mediated by interleukin-8 dependent mechanisms. J Clin Invest 1995;96:107-16.
42. Moss M, Steinberg K, Guidot D, Duhon GF, Treece P, Wolken R, Hudson LD, Parsons PE. Diabetic patients with septic shock have decreased incidence of the acute respiratory distress syndrome (ARDS). Am J Respir Crit Care Med 1997;155:A503.
43. Wayte J, Silva AT, Krausz T, Cohen J. Observations on the role of tumor necrosis factor alpha in a murine model of shock due to Streptococcus pyogenes. Crit Care Med 1993;21:1207-12.
44. Reinhart K, Wiegand-Lohnert C, Grimminger F, Kaul M, Withington S, Treacher D, Eckart J, Willats S, Bouza C, Krausch D, Stockenhuber F, Eiselstein J, Daum L, Kempeni J. Assessment of the safety and efficacy of the monoclonal anti-tumor necrosis factor antibody-fragment, MAK 195F, in patients with sepsis and septic shock: a multicenter, randomized, placebo-controlled, dose-ranging study. Crit Care Med 1996;24:733-42.
45. Hack CE, DeGroot ER, Felt-Bersma RJF, Nuijens JH, Strack Van Schinjndel RJ, Eerenberg-Belmer AJ, Thijs LG, Aarden LA. In plasma levels of interleukin-6 in sepsis. Blood 1989;7:1704-10.
46. Dinarello CA, Gelfland JA, Wolff SM. Anticytokine strategies in the treatment of systemic inflammatory response syndrome. JAMA 1993;269:1829-35.
47. Dellinger RP. Tumor necrosis factor in septic shock and multiple system trauma. Crit Care Med 1997;25:1771-3.
48. Strieter R, Kunkel S, Bone R. Role of tumor necrosis factor-alpha in disease states and inflammation. Crit Care Med 1993;21(suppl):S447-63.
49. Roumen R, Hendriks T, van der Ven-Jongerkrisg J, Nieuwenhuijzen GA, Sauerwein RW, van der Meer JW, Goris RJ. Cytokine patterns in patients after major vascular surgery, hemorrhagic shock, and severe blunt trauma. Relation with subsequent adult respiratory distress syndrome and multiple organ failure. Ann Surg 1993;218:767-76.
50. McClain C, Hill D, Schmidt J, Diehl AM. Cytokines and alcoholic liver disease. Semin Liver Dis 1993;13:170-82.
51. Bell S, Chavali S, Bistrian B, Connolly CA, Utsunomiya T, Forse RA. Dietary fish oil and cytokine and eicosanoid production during human immunodeficiency virus infection. JPEN 1996;20:43-9.
52. Brivet FG, Emilie D, Galanaud P. Pro- and anti-inflammatory cytokines during acute severe pancreatitis: and early and sustained response although unpredictable of death. Parisian Study group on acute pancreatitis. Crit Care Med 1999;27:749-55.
53. Vincent JL, Bakker J, Marecaux G, Schandene L, Kahn RJ, Dupont E. Administration of anti-TNF antibody improves left ventricular function in septic shock patients: Results of a pilot study. Chest 1992;101:810-5.
54. Abraham E, Glauser MP, Butler T, Garbino J, Gelmont D, Laterre PF, Kudsk K, Bruining HA, Otto C, Tobin E, Zwingelstein C, Lesslauer W, Leighton A. p55 tumor necrosis factor receptor fusion protein in the treatment of patients with severe sepsis and septic shock: a randomized controlled multicenter trial. JAMA 1997;277:1531-8.

55. Kushner I. C-reactive protein and the acute phase response. Hosp Pract 1990;25:13-28.
56. Chwals WJ, Fernandez M, Jamie A, Charles BJ, Rushing JT. Detection of postoperative sepsis in infants with the use of metabolic stress monitoring. Arch Surg 1994;129:437-42.
57. Shaw AC. Serum C-reactive protein and neopterin concentrations in patients with viral or bacterial infection. J Clin Pathol 1991;44:596-9.
58. Yentis SM, Soni N, Sheldon J. C-reactive protein as a indicator of resolution of sepsis in the intensive care unit. Inten Care Med 1998;21:602-605.
59. Provoa P, Almeida E, Moreira P, Fernandes A, Mealha R, Aragao A, Sabino H. C-reactive protein as an indicator of sepsis. Inten Care Med 1998;24:1052-1056.
60. Ugarte H, Silva E, Mercan D, De Mendonca A, Vincent JL. Procalcitonin as a marker of infection in the intensive care unit. Crit Care Med 1999;27:498-504.
61. Rau B, Steinbach G, Gansauge F, Mayer JM, Grunert A, Beger HG. The potential role of procalcitonin and interleukin-8 in the prediction of infected necrosis in acute pancreatitis. Gut 1997;41:832-40.
62. Eberhard OK, Langefeld I, Kuse ER, Brunkhorst FM, Kliem V, Schlitt HJ, Pichlmayr R, Koch KM, Brunkhorst R. Procalcitonin in the early phase after renal transplantation-will it add to diagnostic accuracy? Clin Transplant 1998;12:206-211.

Chapter 2

DEFINITIONS: SEPSIS VERSUS SIRS

Jean-Louis Vincent, M.D.
Department of Intensive Care, Erasme Hospital, Free University of Brussels, Brussels Belgium

Introduction

Definitions are an essential and necessary aspect of understanding in all walks of life, from basic language skills to complex scientific reasoning. Definitions serve to provide us with a precise statement of the nature, properties, scope, or essential qualities of a word, or more abstractly, of an event, concept or process. Definitions can be simple or detailed and the degree of definition will depend on its purpose. Importantly, definitions must not be viewed as inflexible, but, rather, must be able to be adapted and adjusted as new information and knowledge becomes available regarding the item in question.

Medicine is an area in which definitions form a cornerstone of basic medical education and diagnosis. With the pace of modern science and research, many areas of medicine are beset by definitions which are vague, imprecise and incomplete. In addition, while certain diseases or syndromes can be clearly and simply defined, in other conditions definitions can be confused, unclear and sometimes unhelpful. Sepsis is one such area where it is easy to get bogged down in terminology and definition, rather than concentrating on the underlying concepts. In this chapter, we will discuss the various definitions and attempt to clear away some of the blurred edges.

Sepsis

The word sepsis originates from the Greek words sepsis meaning to decay and sepein meaning to putrefy. Sepsis, in fact, represents the body's systemic response to severe infection, and is the result of a complex interaction between the host and the invading organism resulting in the release of a myriad of inflammatory mediators. Importantly, it is the presence of an infectious organism which elicits this inflammatory response and infection is therefore implicit in the definition and diagnosis of sepsis. The terms 'infection' and 'sepsis' are often used as synonyms, but their meanings are not the same. Infection is a microbiological event caused by bacteria, fungi, viruses, etc. Sepsis is the systemic response to that infection. Thus, while infection can exist without sepsis, the reverse is not true; genuine sepsis can only be present if there is also an infection (Figure 1). Once sepsis has been diagnosed, septic shock is generally accepted as being the association of sepsis with hypotension (systolic arterial pressure < 90 mmHg, mean arterial pressure < 60 mmHg) requiring vasopressor agents, and signs of tissue hypoperfusion such as increased blood lactate levels, oliguria, altered mentation, etc. (1).

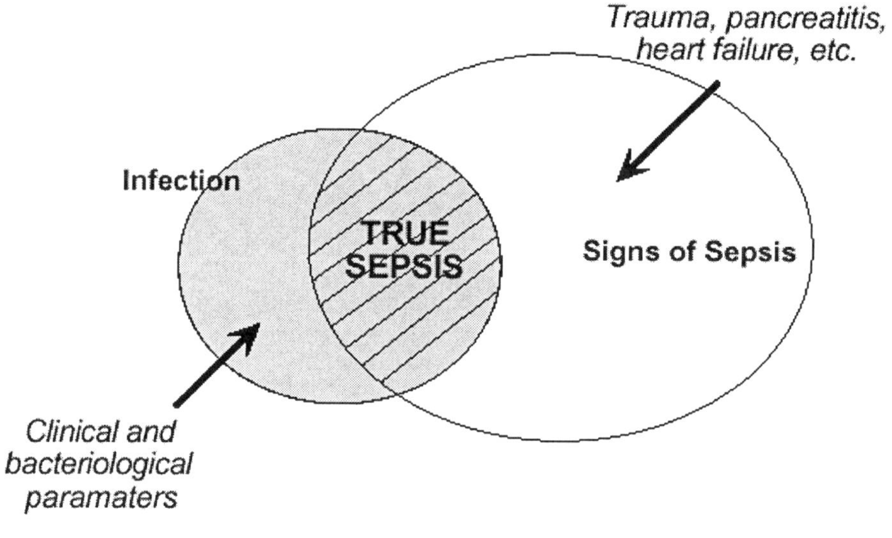

Figure 1. The interrelation between infection and signs of sepsis

The 'problem' with sepsis

The main difficulty with the definition of sepsis is the question of infection. It is certainly true that a 'sepsis-like' syndrome can be present in patients with various disease processes unrelated to the presence of infection, although it may be that in some of these patients translocation of bacteria or bacterial products from the gut (and hence infection of a sort) may be involved (2,3). As discussed above, however, the presence of infection is a prerequisite for a diagnosis of 'true' sepsis. The problem then lies in the identification and diagnosis of infection. Particularly in the intensive care unit (ICU) patient who has already received, or is receiving, antibiotics for one reason or another, and has multiple risk factors for infection and often several concurrent disease processes, infection may be hard to locate. Importantly, bacteremia is not essential for a diagnosis of sepsis. Only about 50% of patients with severe sepsis will have documented bacteremia (4). Repeated careful clinical assessment along with cultures of body fluids and X-ray imaging is necessary to try and identify a source of infection in the patient with suspected sepsis. Even so, some patients will have obvious signs of sepsis and yet the source of infection cannot be demonstrated. This does not, however, necessarily mean that no infection is present, perhaps that we are just unable to find it!

Sepsis is characterized by the presence of a variety of clinical signs, altered biochemical parameters, and typical hemodynamic changes (Table 1). However, many of the so-called 'classical' signs of sepsis are also present in patients without infection. For example, fever is a common feature of sepsis, but is also often present in non-infected ICU patients (5), for example following myocardial infarction or pulmonary embolism, or post-operatively (6). In addition, some patients with sepsis, may show hypothermia which may, in fact, be associated with a worse outcome (7-9). Similarly a raised white cell count is common in sepsis, but again may be caused by other disease processes, and some patients with sepsis will show a reduced white cell count. Thus, none of these signs listed in Table 1 is specific for sepsis.

Table 1: 'Classical' signs of sepsis

Fever (sometimes hypothermia)
Tachycardia
Tachypnea
Elevated cardiac output
Low systemic vascular resistance
Increased cellular metabolism
Increased insulin requirements
Raised (sometimes reduced) white cell count
Increased inflammatory markers: raised C-reactive protein, raised sedimentation rate
Organ dysfunction

Biochemical markers have been proposed as providing more concrete evidence of the presence of sepsis and the list of suggested candidates is long (and growing!) (Table 2). Levels of those cytokines participating in the inflammatory response to infection would seem to be an obvious marker for sepsis. Increased levels of certain cytokines have been well-documented in patients with sepsis and some have been correlated with outcome (10-13). However, as with clinical signs, changes in the levels of cytokines are not specific for sepsis. In addition, increased cytokine levels may be transient and not present at all time points during the course of the disease. For example, tumor necrosis factor (TNF) is certainly raised early in the course of sepsis, but such increases are also found in other conditions including acute pancreatitis (14), trauma (15), myocardial infarction (16), and heart failure (17), and later in the disease process, these levels may fall. The same is seen with other cytokines including interleukin (IL)-6, although this is generally the cytokine which most consistently has raised levels in sepsis. Based on this, the presence of IL-6 levels > 1000pg/ml has been used as an entry criterion for a clinical trial of an anti-TNF antibody therapy (18,19).

Table 2. Some proposed laboratory markers of sepsis

White blood cell count
C-reactive protein (CRP)
Cytokine levels: TNF, IL-6, IL-8, IL-10, TNF receptors, ...
Procalcitonin
Serum amyloid protein
Neopterin
Elastase
Phospholipase A_2
Endothelin-1
Nitrates/nitrites
P-selectin/E-selectin
Prolactin
Lactoferrin
Lipopolysaccharide binding protein

Other markers of inflammation have also been suggested as being of use in the diagnosis of sepsis and some, such as C-reactive protein (CRP), are in common use, particularly in Europe. CRP has been shown to be a useful indicator of the presence of sepsis (20), and more indicative of infection than the white cell count or fever (21). CRP levels > 17 mg/dl have been suggested as providing a means of separating patients with sepsis from those with a non-septic inflammatory response due to trauma (22). Procalcitonin has also been proposed as a marker of infection (23-25), but may be more useful as an indicator of the severity of infection rather than as a marker of the presence of infection per se (26). Various other molecules have been suggested as markers of sepsis including neopterin (27) and elastase (28). However, as with cytokine levels, these are all markers of inflammation rather than infection, and none are specific for sepsis.

SIRS

It is an accepted fact that some patients can present with a clinical picture of sepsis but have no infection; as infection is a prerequisite for a diagnosis of sepsis, these patients could be said to have a 'sepsis-like' syndrome. This is an important differentiation, as antibiotics should not be given to all patients with signs of sepsis, but only to those with clinical and/or bacteriological evidence of infection. The realization that the same inflammatory response seen in sepsis, involving the same cytokines and mediators, could also be seen in other disease processes, led to the creation of the term 'systemic inflammatory response syndrome' (SIRS) (29). This concept was developed by a North-American consensus conference of critical care physicians in an attempt to clarify the definition of patients with a clinical inflammatory response arising from a nonspecific insult, and to create some uniformity in definitions for comparison of groups included in clinical trials of innovative anti-sepsis treatments. According to this definition, a patient has SIRS when at least two of four parameters are present: temperature > 38°C or < 36°C; heart rate > 90 beats per minute; respiratory rate > 20 breaths per minute or PCO_2 < 32 mmHg; white blood cell count >12 x 10^9/l or < 4.0 x 10^9/l. Sepsis, by this definition, was defined as the presence of SIRS in association with a confirmed infectious process; severe sepsis as the presence of sepsis with either hypotension or systemic indications of hypoperfusion; and septic shock as sepsis with hypotension despite fluid resuscitation, and hypoperfusion abnormalities including hyperlactatemia, oliguria and altered mental status.

The 'problem' with SIRS

The concept of SIRS has several problems (30). First, the need for new acronyms is doubtful; the concepts can be adequately explained with existing terminology. Second, SIRS criteria are highly sensitive and most ICU patients and many general ward patients have SIRS (31-34). Indeed, during the course of a normal day, many healthy individuals will have SIRS, for example, when we run to catch a bus and become a little tachypneic and tachycardic. The criteria for sepsis included in the SIRS definition are also more sensitive than most practicing physicians would accept (35). Third, a 'diagnosis' of SIRS provides no actual information regarding the underlying disease process, if any. SIRS indicates the presence of an inflammatory response, but the question can be raised whether SIRS represents a disease process *per se,* or in fact whether patients with SIRS are exhibiting an appropriate physiologic response (36). Indeed, the inflammatory response 'defined' in the SIRS criteria is in fact a beneficial part of the body's normal fight against infection and disease, and a 'diagnosis' of SIRS is in fact no diagnosis at all. Fourth, if used as a diagnostic label, SIRS could potentially remove the incentive to search for infection and delay the start of beneficial antibiotic treatment. Fifth, excessive simplicity can be harmful. Even though SIRS is very sensitive, patients may be suspected of having sepsis on the basis of other abnormalities, such as a high cardiac output, increased CRP, unexplained disseminated intravascular coagulation (DIC) or hyperbilirubinemia. Finally, the high sensitivity of SIRS limits its usefulness as an entry criteria for clinical trials of therapeutic agents in ICU patients although several studies have used it as such. Increasing sensitivity can limit specificity, and particularly in the field of immunomodulatory therapies in sepsis, we are increasingly realizing the importance of appropriately targeting treatments at certain patient groups. Thus the inclusion of all patients with an inflammatory response (i.e., all SIRS patients), even when the degree of response is categorized by severity scores, will likely lead to negative trial results as any beneficial effect in a small subgroup of appropriate patients will be negated by the overall negative effect in the heterogeneous group.

Sepsis versus SIRS

Definitions in sepsis have become somewhat confused as the complexities of the sepsis response have been unraveled. However, the important feature of a definition of sepsis must be that it provides some indication of the underlying pathologic processes, i.e., infection. The basic variables used in the definition of SIRS are non-specific indicators of inflammation which can be present in many disease process including but not exclusive to sepsis. Today, the most important aspect of sepsis, for the physician and patient, is the identification of infection, which can be treated with appropriate antibiotics and removal of the focus of infection where possible. A definition of SIRS may detract from the important search for an infectious process and hence delay treatment. The problem with SIRS is that it has been used as a diagnostic label and yet it carries no pathogenetic information and indeed is merely a description of the presence of an inflammatory process which can be a normal physiologic event or the result of a pathologic disease process. The majority of ICU patients, and indeed many healthy individuals, will exhibit SIRS at some time but this provides no indication as to what treatment if any should be instituted. The presence of an inflammatory response *per se* is not necessarily a negative feature; the underlying cause of the response needs to be ascertained before the need for treatment can be assessed.

CONCLUSIONS

The importance of a diagnosis of sepsis lies in establishing correct treatment for today's patient, and enabling the development and of new treatments for the future. The challenge for the physician faced with a septic patient is not to get diverted by definitions but to locate and identify the underlying causative infection. Sepsis is a complex process and there is no real need to try and simplify it, but rather to better understand the underlying mechanisms involved. While new markers specific for infection rather than inflammation need to be developed, at present physicians must rely on the presence of a number of signs and markers in their diagnosis of sepsis; no one variable alone is sufficient. Importantly every effort must be made to identify the nature and source of infection so that appropriate treatment can be rapidly instituted.

REFERENCES

1. Vincent JL (1994) Sepsis and septic shock: Update on definitions. In: Eyrich K, Sprung C, Reinhart K (eds) Update in Intensive Care and Emergency Medicine. Springer Verlag, Berlin,pp 3-15.
2. Meakins JL, Marshall JC (1989) The gut as the motor of multiple system organ failure. In: Marston A, Buckley GB, Fiddian-Green R (eds) Splanchnic ischemia and multiple organ failure. Edward Arnold Ltd, London,pp 339-348.
3. Niebauer J, Volk HD, Kemp M, et al (1999) Endotoxin and immune activation in chronic heart failure: a prospective cohort study. Lancet 353: 1838-1842.
4. Bone RC, Fisher CJ, Clemmer TP, Slotman GJ, Metz CA, Balk RA (1989) Sepsis syndrome: A valid clinical entity. Crit Care Med 17: 389-393.
5. Circiumaru B, Baldock G, Cohen J (1999) A prospective study of fever in the intensive care unit. Intensive Care Med 25: 668-673.
6. Clarke DE, Kimelman J, Raffin TA (1991) The evaluation of fever in the intensive care unit. Chest 100: 213-220.
7. Clemmer TP, Fisher CJ, Bone RC, Slotman GJ, Metz GA, Thomas FO (1992) Hypothermia in the sepsis syndrome and clinical outcome. Crit Care Med 20: 1395-1401.
8. Brun-Buisson C, Doyon F, Carlet J, et al (1995) Incidence, risk factors, and outcome of severe sepsis and septic shock in adults. A multicenter prospective study in intensive care units. J A M A 274: 968-974.
9. Pittet D, Thievent B, Wenzel RP, Li N, Auckenthaler R, Suter PM (1996) Bedside prediction of mortality from bacteremic sepsis. A dynamic analysis of ICU patients. Am J Respir Crit Care Med 153: 684-693.

10. Calandra T, Baumgartner JD, Grau DG, et al (1990) Prognostic values of tumor necrosis factor/cachectin, interleukin-1, interferon-alpha, and interferon-gamma in the serum of patients with septic shock. J Infect Dis 161: 982-987.
11. Pinsky MR, Vincent JL, Deviere J (1993) Serum cytokine levels in human septic shock : Relation to multiple-systems organ failure and mortality. Chest 103: 565-575.
12. Terregino CA, Lopez BL, Karras DJ, Killian AJ, Arnold GK (2000) Endogenous mediators in emergency department patients with presumed sepsis: are levels associated with progression to severe sepsis and death? Ann Emerg Med 35: 26-34.
13. Gogos CA, Drosou E, Bassaris HP, Skoutelis A (2000) Pro- versus anti-inflammatory cytokine profile in patients with severe sepsis: A marker for prognosis and future therapeutic options. J Infect Dis 181: 176-180.
14. Brivet FG, Emilie D, Galanaud P (1999) Pro- and anti-inflammatory cytokines during acute severe pancreatitis: an early and sustained response, although unpredictable of death. Parisian Study Group on Acute Pancreatitis. Crit Care Med 27: 749-755.
15. Ferguson KL, Taheri P, Rodriguez J, Tonapi V, Cardellio A, Dechert R (1997) Tumor necrosis factor activity increases in the early response to trauma. Acad Emerg Med 4: 1035-1040.
16. Neumann FJ, Ott I, Gawaz M, et al (1995) Cardiac release of cytokines and inflammatory responses in acute myocardial infarction. Circulation 92: 748-755.
17. Vonhof S, Brost B, Stille-Siegener M, Grumbach IM, Kreuzer H, Figulla HR (1998) Monocyte activation in congestive heart failure due to coronary artery disease and idiopathic dilated cardiomyopathy. Int J Cardiol 63: 237-244.
18. Reinhart K, Wiegand-Löhnert C, Grimminger F, et al (1996) Assessment of the safety and efficacy of the monoclonal anti-tumor necrosis factor antibody fragment, MAK195F, in patients with sepsis and septic shock: A multicenter, randomized, placebo-controlled, dose ranging study. Crit Care Med 24: 733-742.
19. Reinhart K, RAMSES Study Group (1998) Treatment of severe sepsis in patients with highly elevated IL-6 levels with anti-TNF monoclonal antibody MAK 195F: The RAMSES study. Crit Care 2: P18 (Abst).
20. Matson A, Soni N, Sheldon J (1991) C-reactive protein as a diagnostic test of sepsis in the critically ill. Anaesth Intensive Care 19: 182-186.
21. Póvoa P, Almeida E, Moreira P, et al (1998) C-reactive protein as an indicator of sepsis. Intensive Care Med 24: 1052-1056.
22. Miller PR, Munn DD, Meredith JW, Chang MC (1999) Systemic inflammatory response syndrome in the trauma intensive care unit: who is infected? J Trauma 47: 1004-1008.
23. Assicot M, Gendrel D, Carsin H, Raymond J, Guilbaud J, Bohoun C (1993) High serum procalcitonin concentration in patients with sepsis and infection. Lancet 341: 515-518.
24. Al-Nawas B, Krammer I, Shah PM (1996) Procalcitonin in diagnosis of severe infections. Eur J Med Res 1: 331-333.
25. Brunkhorst FM, Eberhard OK, Brunkhorst R (1999) Discrimination of infectious and noninfectious causes of early acute respiratory distress syndrome by procalcitonin. Crit Care Med 27: 2172-2176.
26. Ugarte H, Silva E, Mercan D, de Mendonça A, Vincent JL (1999) Procalcitonin as a marker of infection in the intensive care unit. Crit Care Med 27: 498-504.
27. Yao YM, Yu Y, Wang YP, Tian HM, Sheng ZY (1996) Elevated serum neopterin level: its relation to endotoxemia and sepsis in patients with major burns. Eur J Clin Invest 26: 224-230.

28. Bossink AW, Groeneveld AB, Thijs LG (1999) Prediction of microbial infection and mortality in medical patients with fever: plasma procalcitonin, neutrophilic elastase-alpha1- antitrypsin, and lactoferrin compared with clinical variables. Clin Infect Dis 29: 398-407.
29. ACCP-SCCM Consensus Conference (1992) Definitions of sepsis and multiple organ failure and guidelines for the use of innovative therapies in sepsis. Crit Care Med 20: 864-874.
30. Vincent JL (1997) Dear Sirs, I'm sorry to say that I don't like you.. Crit Care Med 25: 372-374.
31. Pittet D, Rangel-Frausto S, Li N, et al (1995) Systemic inflammatory response syndrome, sepsis, severe sepsis and septic shock: incidence, morbidities and outcomes in surgical ICU patients. Intensive Care Med 21: 302-309.
32. Rangel Frausto MS, Pittet D, Costigan M, Hwang T, Davis CS, Wenzel RP (1995) The natural history of the systemic inflammatory response syndrome (SIRS). A prospective study. J A M A 273: 117-123.
33. Salvo I, de Cian W, Musicco M, et al (1995) The Italian SEPSIS study: Preliminary results on the incidence and evolution of SIRS, sepsis, severe sepsis and septic shock. Intensive Care Med 21: S244-S249.
34. Bossink AW, Groeneveld J, Hack CE, Thijs LG (1998) Prediction of mortality in febrile medical patients: How useful are systemic inflammatory response syndrome and sepsis criteria? Chest 113: 1533-1541.
35. Opal SM (1998) The uncertain value of the definition for SIRS. Chest 113: 1442-1443.
36. Marshall J (1997) Both the disposition and the means of cure: "Severe SIRS," "sterile shock," and the ongoing challenge of description. Crit Care Med 25: 1765-1766.

Chapter 3

TOLL-LIKE RECEPTORS

Jérôme Pugin, M.D.
Division of Medical Intensive Care, University Hospital of Geneva, Geneva, Switzerland

Innate immune responses to microbes

Molecular recognition of bacterial, non-self molecules is a critical event in the initiation of innate immune responses. This important function has been conserved throughout evolution from insects to humans (1-4). Several host cell surface receptors mediating this function have been identified. Some of these molecules, such as the mannose receptor, the scavenger receptor and complement receptors bind bacteria and bacterial molecules, enhance the cell's ability to ingest and clear out the invading microbe, but do not mediate cell activation (1, 5). Another class of molecules of the innate immunity is composed of circulating soluble proteins, generally acute phase reactants, which recognize and bind bacteria and bacterial molecules with high affinity. Their function is to opsonize the microbe (lipopolysaccharide (LPS)-binding protein, LBP; soluble CD14, sCD14, complement fractions, C-reactive protein), and to shuttle bacterial molecules such as LPS to cell surface receptors or to high density lipoproteins (LBP, sCD14). Some of these proteins, such as the bactericidal/permeability increasing (BPI) protein, have direct bactericidal activity (1). The third class of molecules of the innate immunity includes cell surface receptors which recognize and bind whole bacteria or conserved bacterial molecules such as LPS. Receptors responding to this definition are CD14 and the newly discovered *Toll-like receptors (TLRs),* reviewed in (2, 4, 6-16). Importantly, engagement of these receptors induces the activation of immune cells with the production of a wide variety of responses including the secretion of cytokines, chemokines, the production of oxygen and nitrogen radicals, pro-coagulants, proteolytic enzymes, etc. Engagement of both these soluble and cellular responses corresponds to the first line of defense, i.e. the innate limb of the immunity, and is aimed at controlling the invading microorganism and eventually killing it. It also generates inflammation, local or systemic depending on the site of the infection. Inadequacy in the magnitude, timing or localization of this response may lead to pathological conditions such as the sepsis syndrome (17, 18).

CD14

CD14, a 55 kDa glycosylphosphatidyl-inositol (GPI) anchored myeloid glycoprotein, was identified in 1990 as an important cell surface receptor binding LPS-LBP complexes (19). Both *in vitro* and *in vivo* studies have demonstrated the critical role of CD14 in the mediation of immune responses to endotoxin (20-23). CD14 was subsequently shown to bind and mediate cell activation in response to several other conserved surface bacterial ligands, such as Gram-positive peptidoglycan, lipoteichoic acid, lipoproteins, and mycobacterial lipoarabinomannan (24). It was proposed that CD14 represented the prototypic example of a "pattern recognition receptor" (3, 24). The soluble form of CD14 (sCD14) is found at micromolar concentrations in serum from mammals including humans. Its role is to bind LPS and other bacterial ligands, and to mediate activation of cells which do not bear CD14, such as endothelial and epithelial cells (25, 26). Since CD14 lacks a transmembrane region (GPI anchoring), it has long been postulated that CD14 should associate with another transmembrane signaling protein to mediate cell responses to endotoxin (23).

Drosophila Toll

An important breakthrough in our understanding of innate immune responses came with the identification of a new class of mammalian type I membrane proteins, the *Toll-like receptors (TLRs)* (27-29). TLRs' ancestor, Toll, was initially isolated and cloned in *Drosophila*, and was shown to carry a dual function in the fly. Toll was shown to be important in the fly's embryogenesis (dorso-ventral patterning) but also in innate immune responses against fungi (30-33). Its intracellular region shared significant homology with the IL-1 receptor 1 (34). Binding of *Drosophila* Toll by its ligand, spätzle, activated a signal transduction pathway homologous to that of the mammalian nuclear-factor kappaB (NFκB) pathway, leading to the production of antifungal peptides (31). Eighteen wheeler (18-wheeler), another *Drosophila* Toll-like receptor with immune function (defense against Gram-negative bacteria) was subsequently identified (35, 36).

Interestingly, proteins homologous to Toll with anti-microbial properties were found in several plants (37-39).

Toll-like receptors

In 1997, Medzhitov et al. cloned the first human homologue of *Drosophila* Toll, human Toll (hToll, known as TLR4 in the most recent nomenclature) (28). A chimeric mutant of hToll (CD4 ectodomain and hToll intracellular domain) was found to constitutively activate the NF-κB pathway when transfected to human cells (28). Rapidly, several other human Toll-like receptors were identified from deposited DNA sequences of unknown function, and named TLR1 to TLR5 (27, 29). An additional mammalian member of the TLR family was subsequently identified, TLR6 (40). The amino acid sequence of human TLR6 (hTLR6) is most similar to that of hTLR1. Several other members of this family have been cloned by private companies (15). TLRs were mapped to different chromosomes: chromosome 5 for TLR1 and TLR6, long arm of chromosome 4 for TLR2 and TLR3, chromosome 9 for TLR4, and chromosome 1 for TLR5 (29). RP105, a murine B-cell Toll-like receptor, had actually been cloned before this emerging family of receptors was identified (41, 42). The cell distribution and chromosome location are indicated in Table 1.

Table 1. Cell and chromosome distribution of TLRs

Receptor:	*Expressed in:*	*Chromosome*	*Reference*
TLR1	"Ubiquitous", all leukocytes	5	(15)
TLR2	Blood mononuclear cells	4	(15, 43)
	Gut epithelial cells (mRNA)		(44)
TLR3	"Specific ?", dendritic cells	4	(15)
TLR4	Monocytes, macrophages, neutrophils	9	(15, 45)
	Kupffer cells		(46)
	B-cell lymphocytes		(45, 47)
	Endothelial cells		(48, 49)
	Gut epithelial cells (mRNA)		(44)
	Lung epithelial cells		(50)
TLR5	Lung and liver (murine)	1	(51)
	Myeloid cells		(15)
TLR6	Spleen, thymus, ovary and lung	5	(40)

Similarly to the *Drosophila* Toll, mammalian TLRs show significant homology in their cytoplasmic domain with that of the receptors of the IL-

1R/IL-18R superfamily, and with the intracytoplasmic adaptor molecule MyD88 (52). This domain is now known as the TLR/IL-1R (TIR) domain. The extracellular portion of TLRs is striking by its conserved leucin-reach repeats (LRRs), a feature that is also present in CD14, and which has been associated with protein-protein interaction. Interestingly, this ectodomain appears to be highly polymorphic among different individuals, both in humans and in mice, whereas the intracellular region of TLR4 is far less polymorphic (14, 53). Mutations in this domain result in either gain-of-function (active TLR4 mutant) (28) or loss-of-function (inactive TLR2 mutant) (54). Close to the transmembrane region a cystein-rich domain of unknown significance is also present. A schematic view of the TLRs/IL-1/IL-18 receptor superfamily is shown in Fig. 1.

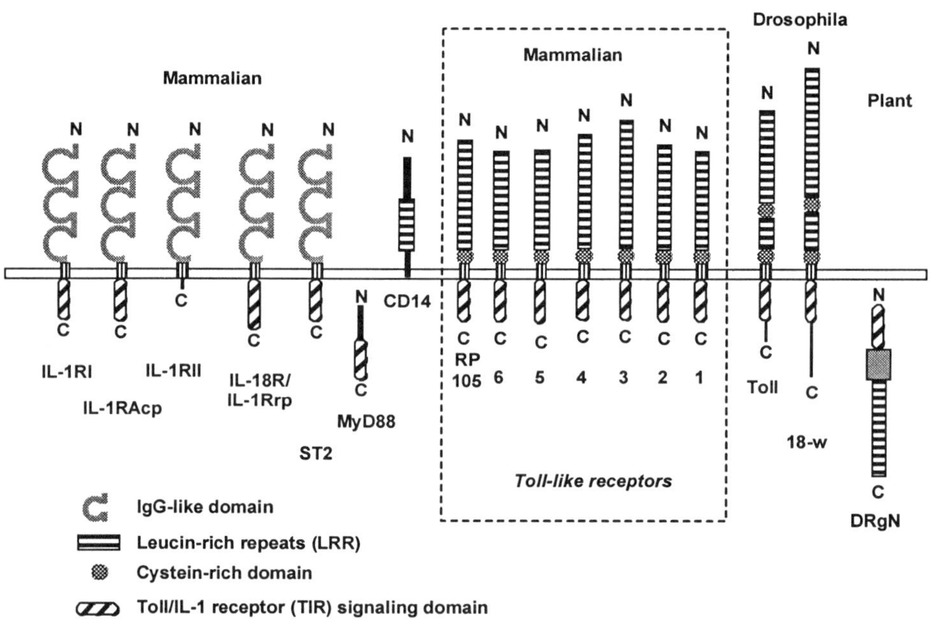

Figure 1. The Toll-like/IL-1 receptor superfamily

TLR2

In 1998, Yang et al., and Kirschning et al. independently identified TLR2 as a potential signal-transducing LPS receptor chain (54, 55). These authors showed that TLR2 conferred responsiveness to LPS when transfected to unresponsive human 293 cells. LPS responses were enhanced by the presence of LBP and CD14 in its membrane or soluble form. TLR2 co-immunoprecipitated with CD14 in cells expressing both molecules (43). It is however important to realize that micromolar concentrations of LPS were necessary to induce a cell response in 293 cells, whereas mouse or human macrophages respond to nanomolar or subnanomolar concentrations of endotoxin. Similarly to CD14, it was subsequently recognized that TLR2 mediated cell activation in response to other bacterial molecules such as peptidoglycan, lipoteichoic acid, lipoarabinomannan, and lipoproteins from *M.tuberculosis*, *B.burgdorferi, and Mycoplasma.* (56-63). This promiscuity of TLR2 for a wide variety of bacterial molecules certainly implies that it corresponds like CD14 to the definition of a pattern recognition receptor (64). TLR2 also mediates responses to several different whole Gram-positive bacteria, including *S.aureus, S.pneumoniae, B.subtilis, L.monocytogenes*, as well as *M.tuberculosis, M.avium, B.burgdorferi* (61, 64). TLR2 also seems to mediate "pro-apoptotic" signals in response to bacterial lipoproteins, but not in response to endotoxin (56). TLR2 was found to be expressed at the surface of peripheral blood mononuclear cells, mainly CD14(+) monocytes and a subset of B lymphocytes (43). TLR2 mRNA expression is increased by the treatment of monocytic cells with LPS (54). However, information is still lacking as to its real participation in LPS-dependent blood leukocyte or macrophage activation. Human primary microvascular endothelial cells express both TLR2 (low levels) and TLR4 (higher levels) (48, 49), and are likely to signal through TLR4 in response to LPS (48). However whether TLR4 represents the receptor for soluble CD14 (25, 65) remains to be determined.

TLR4

In parallel to the studies with TLR2, important work from different groups indicated that TLR4 may actually be the crucial molecule mediating transmembrane LPS signaling. Various approaches led to this conclusion. First, and most important, came the demonstration that the *lps* gene in the well-characterized C3H/HeJ LPS hyporesponsive mouse strain was indeed a mutated version of TLR4. The genetic defect was first mapped in the region of the TLR4 gene (66). Quickly thereafter, it was demonstrated that TLR4 from these mice carried a single base pair mutation changing a proline into a histidine residue in the TIR domain of TLR4 (67, 68). Importantly, this proline is highly conserved among species and is present in all TLRs, except for TLR3. C57BL/10ScCr mice which are also resistant to the effects of LPS were shown to carry a null mutation of TLR4 (67 , 68). Confirmation of the central role of TLR4 came with the demonstration that an engineered targeted gene disruption of mouse TLR4 induced a strong resistance to endotoxin (69). Work by Takeushi et al. demonstrates that whereas mice with a TLR4 gene disruption are highly resistant to LPS, the same mice with a TLR2 k.o. gene were perfectly responsive to LPS, but were deficient in their response to Gram-positive cell wall components (63). Additional work from Chow et al. indicated that transfection of TLR4 into human LPS unresponsive cells conferred endotoxin responsiveness (70). Further evidence for a major role of TLR4 came from studies with blocking monoclonal antibodies against human TLR4. It was shown that such antibodies abrogated LPS-induced TNF production in peripheral blood mononuclear cells (71). Moreover, it was also shown that Chinese hamster ovary (CHO) cells which naturally carry a null allele for TLR2 are capable of responding to endotoxin, indicating that TLR2 is not essential for LPS responses, at least in this CHO fibroblast model (72). Taken together, these important data indicate that, at least in mice, TLR4 is the dominant, if not the sole signaling molecule mediating LPS responses. Elegant work from the groups of Golenbock and Beutler also indicate that TLR4 may well directly interact with the its ligand, LPS (53, 73). They utilized the fact that murine and human mouse myeloid cells, both responsive to LPS, differentially responded to a deacylated LPS analogue: lipid IVa or LA-14-PP. Mouse and hamster cells respond to this compound where human cells are resistant. Using cross-species transfection experiments of human and mouse or hamster TLR4 genes, investigators from both groups showed that the responsiveness to lipid IVa was exclusively carried by the rodent TLR4 molecule. This indicated an exquisite specificity of murine TLR4 for this modified LPS molecule and strongly suggested a direct interaction between LPS with TLR4. This was somewhat corroborated by Kawasaki et al. who showed that TLR4-MD-2 complexes mediated the specific taxol activation of murine cells (74). However, a direct biochemical evidence of an association between TLR4 and LPS, such as that shown between CD14 and LPS (75), is still lacking. This biochemical interaction may be difficult to demonstrate since it is anticipated that TLR4 is a low-affinity receptor and expressed at low levels on the surface of myeloid cells (14). Therefore the exact sequence of events of LPS transmembrane signaling can only be speculative. Two models seem to emerge: 1) LBP transfers LPS monomers to its major acceptor molecule, CD14. The function of the latter molecule, besides internalization (76), might be to concentrate its ligand at the surface of the cell to allow ligation of LPS or the ternary complex (LPS/LBP/CD14) with a low affinity/abundance signaling molecule (TLR4). 2) LPS ligation to CD14 induces somehow a proteolytic cleavage of (a) molecule(s) near or at the membrane, and by analogy to Drosophila spätzle, it is the binding of the protein product to TLR4 that sends the signal to the interior of the cell (11). Supporting this are the findings by Ding et al. that a natural protein inhibitor (secretory leukocyte protease inhibitor) interferes with LPS functions in macrophages, and the fact that LPS induces such a cascade of proteolytic enzymes in *Limulus* (11, 77).

Non-signaling functions of TLRs

Recent evidence suggests that TLR4 may discriminate LPS from other phospholipid ligands (71). This may be relevant since CD14 was earlier shown to bind phosphoinositides and mediate cell uptake of these endogenous molecules. CD14 also binds phosphatidylserine, a molecule expressed at the surface of apoptotic cells and is therefore implicated in the clearance of apoptotic bodies (78). Whether TLRs participate in these functions remains to be determined. Other important functions of CD14 are the clearance of LPS from the extracellular milieu (76), essentially for detoxification, and the uptake of Gram-negative bacteria (79). In work from Underhill et al. it was shown that a signaling dominant-negative form of TLR2 did not block yeast particle internalization (80). However, our knowledge on a putative role of TLRs in the uptake process of bacteria and bacterial products such as endotoxin remains very fragmental. A puzzling report by Frantz et al. shows that TLR4 is upregulated in myocytes from failing heart both in humans and in a murine model (81). The exact relevance of this finding is unknown, but it may be speculated that TLRs also participate in the regulation of some tissue functions in pathological conditions. Finally, it was recently proposed that heat shock protein 60 (HSP60) binds TLR4, and competes with LPS for signaling (82). HSP60's protein sequence, like TLRs, has been highly conserved during the evolution. It is displayed at the cell surface and released during cell necrosis, and may actually nicely link with the work previously described on failing myocardium. This is also an indication that TLRs, like CD14, may have some important endogenous ligands.

Regulation of TLR4 expression

A preliminary characterization of the promoter sequence of human TLR4 has recently been published by Rehli et al. (45). Interestingly, the 75 base pairs directly upstream of the initiation codon of the TLR4 gene carry all the promoter activity, as demonstrated in a classical luciferase reporter gene assay. This 5' region contains the consensus sequences for the myeloid cell-specific PU.1 transcription factor (also present in the promoter region of CD14) and a γ-interferon (γIFN) response factor (45). Although little is known on the modulation of TLR4 protein *in vitro* and *in vivo*, it can be anticipated that the modulation of its level of expression by γIFN might be very relevant. It has indeed been shown for a long time that the treatment of myeloid cells with γIFN conferred or dramatically increased cell responsiveness to LPS. Interestingly, the importance of γIFN in enhancing TLR4-dependent effects was already clearly delineated by the group of Janeway in their initial report on this molecule, known at the time as hToll (28). Another hint as to the importance of the level of expression of TLR4 in the regulation of myeloid cell responses to LPS comes from the work of Nomura et al. (83). These authors have correlated endotoxin tolerance with the downregulation of surface TLR4 expression. In the same line, it was recently shown that TLR2 and TLR4 were targets for monocyte deactivation by IL-4 (84). Finally, the blockade of TLR4 in mouse macrophages using a monoclonal antibody anti-TLR4-MD2 complex (see below) blunted TNF secretion by these cells in response to LPS (47).

MD molecules

Interestingly, two of the TLRs are co-expressed with "MD" molecules. This is the case for the murine B-cell RP105 TLR which is co-expressed with MD-1, a murine analogue of chicken MD-1, a *v-myb*-regulated gene. MD-1 seems to be required for efficient RP105 surface expression (85, 86). Even more interesting is its analogue MD-2 which was co-purified with TLR4 by the group of Miyake. In this case, MD-2 is not important for TLR4 expression, but is rather essential for TLR4-dependent LPS-activation of cells (87). MD-2 is a soluble protein, i.e. lacks a transmembrane domain, is exteriorized by the cell but somehow remains attached to TLR4. When co-expressed with TLR4, it confers cell responsiveness to subnanomolar concentrations of LPS (87). Based on the reactivity of an anti-TLR4 monoclonal antibody, a recent study by the group of Miyake strongly suggests that MD-2 binding to TLR4 induces a conformational change to TLR4, which might represent the molecular basis for the enhancement of LPS responses by MD-2 (83).

TLR5

The mouse TLR5 cDNA was recently cloned and TLR5 gene mapped to chromosome 1, in a position known to carry the susceptibility to Salmonella typhymurium by the MOLF/Ei mouse strain (51). Murine TLR5 shows an 81% homology with the human TLR5 gene, ~40 % with the other TLRs, and is mainly expressed in the liver and the lung. Infection of MOLF/Ei mice is associated with decreased expression of TLR5 in the liver. Further studies may show evidence for a direct implication of TLR5 in this phenotypic trait, and link TLR5 with the response to Gram-negative infections. Although LPS responses may be attributed to TLR4, particular attention should be paid to the other members of the TLR family. It could be demonstrated that, despite profound defects in LPS responses (63, 67-69), TLR4-deficient mice cope pretty well with severe bacterial infections, in particular with those caused by Gram-negative bacteria. Some other TLRs (or other molecules of the innate immunity) must be implicated in the defense against bacteria and other microbial pathogens.

Reconciling TLR2 and TLR4 functions

Whereas it can be acknowledged that the breakthrough of finding a first function to a TLR came from the work with TLR2 (54, 55), it can also reasonably be stated that TLR2 finds its major function in initiating innate immune responses to non-LPS bacterial ligands, such as peptidoglycan and lipoproteins. Transfection of the human TLR2 gene confers LPS responsiveness to human cell lines not expressing TLR4. However, the amount of LPS required to activate the cells is far from physiological. TLR4 certainly carries the function of the major LPS signaling molecule. The strongest and almost unequivocal evidence for this comes from genetic studies in mice. Such compelling evidence is still lacking in humans, where the situation might actually be slightly different. For example, as stated above, the ligand specificity of TLR4 is different in humans and rodents (see above the case for taxol and lipid IVa), and this may also be true for TLR2. The cell type studied might also be important to define TLR-dependent responses. TLR2 has also been shown to act as a "sensing" mechanism for yeast and Gram-positive particles. This receptor accompanies ingested pathogens from the cell surface to particle-containing phagosomes, and signals when it has "sensed" a non-self intruder (80). A similar behavior of pathogen recognition has not yet been described with other TLRs. Putative TLR functions are summarized in Table 2.

Table 2. Known agonists and functions of TLRs

	Receptor:	*Agonist(s):*	*Implicated in:*	*Ref.*
Drosophila:	*Toll*	spätzle	ontogenesis, defense against fungal infection	(31, 32)
	18-wheeler	?	ontogenesis, defense against Gram-negative infection	(35, 36)
Plants:	*N* (tobacco)		defense against mosaic virus	
	L6 (Flax)		defense against fungi	
	RPP5 (arabidopsis)		defense against fungi	(37-39)
Mammals:	***TLR1***	?	?	
	TLR2	PG, LTA, LAM, lipoproteins	defense against Gram-positive bacterial and mycobacterial infection	(56-59, 61-63, 73, 80, 88-90)
		Lipoproteins	apoptosis	(56)
	TLR3	?	dendritic cells biology ?	(15)
	TLR4	LPS	cell response to endotoxin	(63, 67-71, 89, 91)
		phospholipids	apoptosis ? PLs uptake ?	(71)
		taxol	cell responses to taxol	(74)
		HSP60	tissue necrosis ?	(82)
			TLR4 co-expressed with MD-2	(47, 87)
	TLR5	?	defense against Salmonella ?	(51)
	TLR6	?	activation of NF-kB	(40)
	RP105	?	murine B-cells expression, activation of NF-kB	(42, 92)
			co-expressed with MD-1	(85, 86)

Abbreviations: LPS, lipopolysaccharide, endotoxin ; LTA, lipoteichoic acid ; PG, peptidoglycan ; LAM, lipoarabinomannan; PL, phospholipids.

Signaling *via* Toll-like receptors

Given the similarity in their intracytoplasmic domains, it could rapidly be demonstrated that TLRs and IL-1R/IL-18R shared a common intracellular activation pathway. Similarly to IL-1-dependent signaling, activated TLR2 and TLR4 recruit the adaptor molecule MyD88, and IL-1R-associated kinases (IRAKs), which activate tumor necrosis factor receptor-associated factor 6 (TRAF6), and the "common" NF-κB pathway *via* NIK, and IκB kinases (IKKs) (37, 43, 49, 93-97). As shown in deletion studies, the terminal portion of the cytoplasmic domain of TLRs seems critical for the signaling function (55). The natural C3H/HeJ P712H mutation points at this critical proline residue in TLR4 certainly indicates that this residue is important for the signaling function. The same residue is found at the same position in human and mouse genes in all but TLR3 Toll-like receptors, in the middle of a stretch of ~ 30 highly conserved residues (67). Mutation in this residue generates a dominant negative molecule as shown elegantly with mouse TLR2 by Underhill et al., and blocks TLR2-dependent signaling (80). Activation of mitogen-activated protein kinases (MAPK) also occurs in a MyD88/IRAK-dependent pathway, downstream of MyD88 and IRAK (97), but upstream of TRAF6 (98) (Fig. 2). The molecules linking IRAK and the MAPKK remain to be identified. However it is possible that, by analogy to the IL-1-dependent signaling pathway, small GTP-binding proteins such as Rac-1 and cdc42 might be the "missing link". TAK-1, a MAPKKK has also been implicated in the LPS-induced signaling pathway mediated by both TLR-2 and TLR4 (99). Work with dominant negative mutants of MyD88, IRAK, TRAF6, and NIK have demonstrated the likely implication of these enzymes in the signal transduction pathway dependent on TLR2 (43). However, the unequivocal demonstration that this MyD88/IRAK/TRAF-6 pathway was critical for LPS activation of cells came again from gene "knock out" experiments of the proximal enzymes of the signaling cascade. The targeted disruption of the MyD88 gene resulted in the resistance of mice to endotoxin-related lethality, and these mice did not produce pro-inflammatory cytokines in response to LPS (100). Surprisingly, whereas macrophages and B-lymphocytes from these animals could not be activated by IL-1 and IL-18, LPS still induced a delayed but robust response in terms of NF-κB and MAPK activation (100). The gene knock-out of IRAK-1 showed a quasi identical phenotype as that of the MyD88 k.o. The IRAK-1 k.o. mouse was resistant to an endotoxin challenge, although less than its MyD88 k.o. littermates, and IRAK -/- macrophages showed a marked impairment in LPS responses (97). As with MyD88, the absence of IRAK had dramatic effects on LPS-dependent lethality and gene transcription, however the genetic defect only slightly decreased MAPK activation (ERK2, JNK and p38) (97). A schematic and speculative view of TLR4-dependent cell activation is presented in Fig. 2.

Toll-like receptors and sepsis

The studies discussed above clearly indicate that TLR2, TLR4 and MD-2 are critical molecules for the recognition of bacterial pathogens and for mounting a rapid and efficient immune response. It can therefore be anticipated that modifications in their level of expression or alteration in their sequence/structure, acquired or inherited, will affect innate immune response to microorganisms, and therefore influence local and systemic responses such as those observed during the sepsis syndrome. It is expected that mutations in TLR4 will be identified in patients prone to develop sepsis (14). The report by Kuhns et al. of a patient with severe bacterial infections and a selective defect in LPS and IL-1-dependent activation should prompt

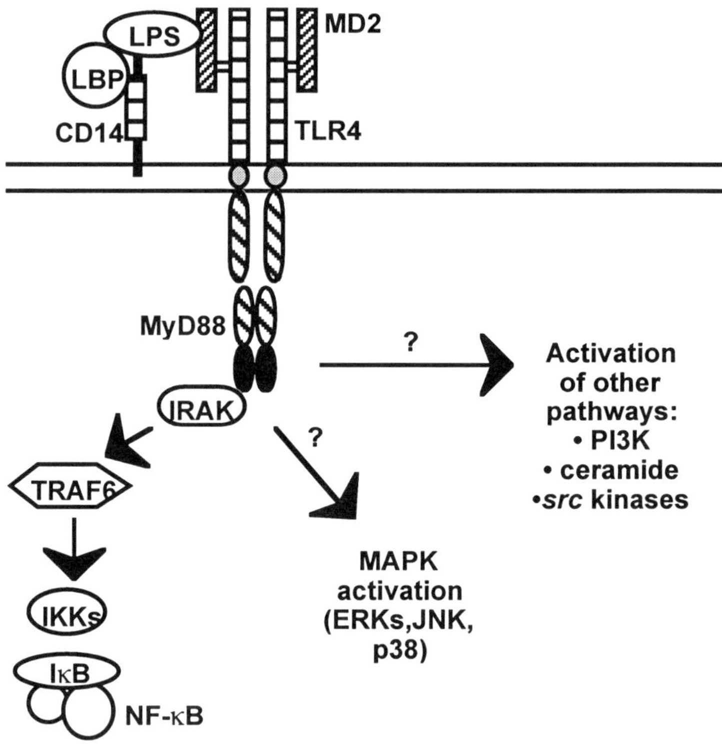

Figure 2. Schematic representation of TLR4-dependent signaling pathway. Abbreviations: LPS, lipopolysaccharide; LBP, lipopolysaccharide-binding protein; IRAK, IL-1 receptor-associated kinase; TRAF6, TNF receptor associated factor 6; IKKs, IκB kinases; NF-κB, nuclear factor-κB; MAPK, mitogen-activated protein kinase; PI3K, PI3 kinase.

investigators to sequence kinases of the common signaling pathway in that particular patient (101). This finding also tells us that polymorphic variations in MyD88, IRAK and TRAK6 genes may well turn out to be important in defining levels of host responses to infection and in the susceptibility to the sepsis syndrome.

Conclusions

Mammalian Toll-like receptors belong to an important and emerging family of receptors of the innate immunity, and have been conserved throughout evolution. Some of them (TLR2 and TLR4) support transmembrane signaling in response to bacterial molecules, and initiate an intracellular cascade of activation of second messengers leading to the transcription of numerous inflammatory genes. They share a pathway common to that of the receptors for IL-1 and IL-18. Additional work is needed 1) to define precise interaction between TLRs and their bacterial ligands; 2) to identify potential endogenous ligands; 3) to define the function of other TLRs; and 4) to test the relevance of TLRs in primary human cells and in diseases.

REFERENCES

1. Fearon DT, Locksley RM. The instructive role of innate immunity in the acquired immune response. Science 1996;272:50-3.
2. Hoffmann JA, Kafatos FC, Janeway CA, Ezekowitz RA. Phylogenetic perspectives in innate immunity. Science 1999;284:1313-8.
3. Janeway CA, Jr. The immune system evolved to discriminate infectious nonself from noninfectious self. Immunol Today 1992;13:11-6.
4. Janeway CA, Jr., Medzhitov R. Introduction: the role of innate immunity in the adaptive immune response. Semin Immunol 1998;10:349-50.
5. Bendelac A, Fearon DT. Innate immunity. Receptors and effectors of innate immunity. Curr Opinion Immunol 2000;12:11-12.
6. Ingalls RR, Heine H, Lien E, Yoshimura A, Golenbock D. Lipopolysaccharide recognition, CD14, and lipopolysaccharide receptors. Infect Dis Clin North Am 1999;13:341-53, vii.
7. Kopp EB, Medzhitov R. The Toll-receptor family and control of innate immunity. Curr Opin Immunol 1999;11:13-8.
8. Qureshi ST, Gros P, Malo D. Host resistance to infection: genetic control of lipopolysaccharide responsiveness by TOLL-like receptor genes. Trends Genet 1999;15:291-4.
9. Ulevitch RJ. Endotoxin opens the Tollgates to innate immunity. Nat Med 1999;5:144-5.
10. Vogel G. Fly development genes lead to immune find. Science 1998;281:1942-4.
11. Wright SD. Toll, a new piece in the puzzle of innate immunity. J Exp Med 1999;189:605-9.
12. O'Neill LA, Dinarello CA. The IL-1 receptor/toll-like receptor superfamily: crucial receptors for inflammation and host defense. Immunol Today 2000;21:206-209.
13. Beutler B. Endotoxin, toll-like receptor 4, and the afferent limb of innate immunity. Curr Opin Microbiol 2000;3:23-8.
14. Beutler B. Tlr4: central component of the sole mammalian LPS sensor. Curr Opin Immunol 2000;12:20-6.
15. Muzio M, Polentarutti N, Bosisio D, Prahladan MK, Mantovani A. Toll-like receptors: a growing family of immune receptors that are differentially expressed and regulated by different leukocytes. J Leukoc Biol 2000;67:450-6.
16. Muzio M, Mantovani A. Toll-like receptors. Microbes Infect 2000;2:251-5.
17. Pugin J. Bacteremia, sepsis and shock. Intensive Care Med 1994;20:92-3.
18. Pugin J. Sepsis and the immune response. Intensive Care Med 1999;25:1027-8.

19. Wright SD, Ramos RA, Tobias PS, Ulevitch RJ, Mathison JC. CD14, a receptor for complexes of lipopolysaccharide (LPS) and LPS binding protein. Science 1990;249:1431-3.
20. Leturcq DJ, Moriarty AM, Talbott G, Winn RK, Martin TR, Ulevitch RJ. Antibodies against CD14 protect primates from endotoxin-induced shock. J Clin Invest 1996;98:1533-8.
21. Pugin J, Ulevitch RJ, Tobias PS. Activation of endothelial cells by endotoxin: direct versus indirect pathways and the role of CD14. Prog Clin Biol Res 1995;392:369-73.
22. Schimke J, Mathison J, Morgiewicz J, Ulevitch RJ. Anti-CD14 mAb treatment provides therapeutic benefit after in vivo exposure to endotoxin. Proc Natl Acad Sci U S A 1998;95:13875-80.
23. Ulevitch RJ, Dunn DL, Fink MP, Taylor CE. Endotoxin-related intracellular pathways: implications for therapeutic intervention. Shock 1996;6:1-2.
24. Pugin J, Heumann ID, Tomasz A, Kravchenko VV, Akamatsu Y, Nishijima M, et al. CD14 is a pattern recognition receptor. Immunity 1994;1:509-16.
25. Pugin J, Schurer-Maly CC, Leturcq D, Moriarty A, Ulevitch RJ, Tobias PS. Lipopolysaccharide activation of human endothelial and epithelial cells is mediated by lipopolysaccharide-binding protein and soluble CD14. Proc Natl Acad Sci U S A 1993;90:2744-8.
26. Pugin J, Ulevitch RJ, Tobias PS. A critical role for monocytes and CD14 in endotoxin-induced endothelial cell activation. J Exp Med 1993;178:2193-200.
27. Chaudhary PM, Ferguson C, Nguyen V, Nguyen O, Massa HF, Eby M, et al. Cloning and characterization of two Toll/Interleukin-1 receptor-like genes TIL3 and TIL4: evidence for a multi-gene receptor family in humans. Blood 1998;91:4020-7.
28. Medzhitov R, Preston-Hurlburt P, Janeway CA, Jr. A human homologue of the Drosophila Toll protein signals activation of adaptive immunity. Nature 1997;388:394-7.
29. Rock FL, Hardiman G, Timans JC, Kastelein RA, Bazan JF. A family of human receptors structurally related to Drosophila Toll. Proc Natl Acad Sci U S A 1998;95:588-93.
30. Lemaitre B, Meister M, Govind S, Georgel P, Steward R, Reichhart JM, et al. Functional analysis and regulation of nuclear import of dorsal during the immune response in Drosophila. Embo J 1995;14:536-45.
31. Lemaitre B, Nicolas E, Michaut L, Reichhart JM, Hoffmann JA. The dorsoventral regulatory gene cassette spatzle/Toll/cactus controls the potent antifungal response in Drosophila adults. Cell 1996;86:973-83.
32. Lemaitre B, Reichhart JM, Hoffmann JA. Drosophila host defense: differential induction of antimicrobial peptide genes after infection by various classes of microorganisms. Proc Natl Acad Sci U S A 1997;94:14614-9.
33. Meister M, Lemaitre B, Hoffmann JA. Antimicrobial peptide defense in Drosophila. Bioessays 1997;19:1019-26.
34. Gay NJ, Keith FJ. Drosophila Toll and IL-1 receptor. Nature 1991;351:355-6.
35. Eldon E, Kooyer S, D'Evelyn D, Duman M, Lawinger P, Botas J, et al. The Drosophila 18 wheeler is required for morphogenesis and has striking similarities to Toll. Development 1994;120:885-99.
36. Williams MJ, Rodriguez A, Kimbrell DA, Eldon ED. The 18-wheeler mutation reveals complex antibacterial gene regulation in Drosophila host defense. Embo J 1997;16:6120-30.

37. O'Neill LA, Greene C. Signal transduction pathways activated by the IL-1 receptor family: ancient signaling machinery in mammals, insects, and plants. J Leukoc Biol 1998;63:650-7.
38. Parker JE, Coleman MJ, Szabo V, Frost LN, Schmidt R, van der Biezen EA, et al. The Arabidopsis downy mildew resistance gene RPP5 shares similarity to the toll and interleukin-1 receptors with N and L6. Plant Cell 1997;9:879-94.
39. Ellis JG, Lawrence GJ, Luck JE, Dodds PN. Identification of regions in alleles of the Flax rust resistance gene *L* that determine differences in gene-for-gene specificity. Plant Cell 1999;11:495-506.
40. Takeuchi O, Kawai T, Sanjo H, Copeland NG, Gilbert DJ, Jenkins NA, et al. TLR6: A novel member of an expanding toll-like receptor family. Gene 1999;231:59-65.
41. Miura Y, Miyake K, Yamashita Y, Shimazu R, Copeland NG, Gilbert DJ, et al. Molecular cloning of a human RP105 homologue and chromosomal localization of the mouse and human RP105 genes (Ly64 and LY64). Genomics 1996;38:299-304.
42. Miyake K, Yamashita Y, Ogata M, Sudo T, Kimoto M. RP105, a novel B cell surface molecule implicated in B cell activation, is a member of the leucine-rich repeat protein family. J Immunol 1995;154:3333-40.
43. Yang RB, Mark MR, Gurney AL, Godowski PJ. Signaling events induced by lipopolysaccharide-activated toll-like receptor 2. J Immunol 1999;163:639-43.
44. Cario E, Rosenberg IM, Brandwein SL, Beck PL, Reinecker HC, Podolsky DK. Lipopolysaccharide activates distinct signaling pathways in intestinal epithelial cell lines expressing Toll-like receptors. J Immunol 2000;164:966-72.
45. Rehli M, Poltorak A, Schwarzfischer L, Krause SW, Andreesen R, Beutler B. PU.1 and interferon consensus sequence-binding protein regulate the myeloid expression of the human toll-like receptor 4 gene. J Biol Chem 2000;275:9773-81.
46. Su GL, Klein RD, Aminlari A, Zhang HY, Steinstraesser L, Alarcon WH, et al. Kupffer cell activation by lipopolysaccharide in rats: role for lipopolysaccharide binding protein and toll-like receptor 4. Hepatology 2000;31:932-6.
47. Akashi S, Shimazu R, Ogata H, Nagai Y, Takeda K, Kimoto M, et al. Cutting edge: cell surface expression and lipopolysaccharide signaling via the toll-like receptor 4-MD-2 complex on mouse peritoneal macrophages. J Immunol 2000;164:3471-5.
48. Faure E, Equils O, Sieling PA, Thomas L, Zhang FX, Kirschning CJ, et al. Bacterial lipopolysaccharide activates NF-kappaB through toll-like receptor 4 (TLR-4) in cultured human dermal endothelial cells. Differential expression of tlr-4 and tlr-2 in endothelial cells. J Biol Chem 2000;275:11058-63.
49. Zhang FX, Kirschning CJ, Mancinelli R, Xu XP, Jin Y, Faure E, et al. Bacterial lipopolysaccharide activates nuclear factor-kappaB through interleukin-1 signaling mediators in cultured human dermal endothelial cells and mononuclear phagocytes. J Biol Chem 1999;274:7611-4.
50. Diamond G, Legarda D, Ryan LK. The innate immune response of the respiratory epithelium. Immunol Rev 2000;173:27-38.
51. Sebastiani G, Leveque G, Lariviere L, Laroche L, Skamene E, Gros P, et al. Cloning and characterization of the murine toll-like receptor 5 (Tlr5) gene: sequence and mRNA expression studies in salmonella-susceptible MOLF/Ei mice [In Process Citation]. Genomics 2000;64:230-40.
52. Hultmark D. Macrophage differentiation marker MyD88 is a member of the Toll/IL-1 receptor family. Biochem Biophys Res Commun 1994;199:144-6.

53. Poltorak A, Ricciardi-Castagnoli P, Citterio S, Beutler B. Physical contact between lipopolysaccharide and toll-like receptor 4 revealed by genetic complementation. Proc Natl Acad Sci U S A 2000;97:2163-7.
54. Yang RB, Mark MR, Gray A, Huang A, Xie MH, Zhang M, et al. Toll-like receptor-2 mediates lipopolysaccharide-induced cellular signalling. Nature 1998;395:284-8.
55. Kirschning CJ, Wesche H, Merrill Ayres T, Rothe M. Human toll-like receptor 2 confers responsiveness to bacterial lipopolysaccharide. J Exp Med 1998;188:2091-7.
56. Aliprantis AO, Yang RB, Mark MR, Suggett S, Devaux B, Radolf JD, et al. Cell activation and apoptosis by bacterial lipoproteins through toll- like receptor-2. Science 1999;285:736-9.
57. Brightbill HD, Libraty DH, Krutzik SR, Yang RB, Belisle JT, Bleharski JR, et al. Host defense mechanisms triggered by microbial lipoproteins through toll-like receptors. Science 1999;285:732-6.
58. Hirschfeld M, Kirschning CJ, Schwandner R, Wesche H, Weis JH, Wooten RM, et al. Cutting edge: inflammatory signaling by Borrelia burgdorferi lipoproteins is mediated by toll-like receptor 2. J Immunol 1999;163:2382-6.
59. Means TK, Lien E, Yoshimura A, Wang S, Golenbock DT, Fenton MJ. The CD14 ligands lipoarabinomannan and lipopolysaccharide differ in their requirement for Toll-like receptors. J Immunol 1999;163:6748-55.
60. Means TK, Wang S, Lien E, Yoshimura A, Golenbock DT, Fenton MJ. Human toll-like receptors mediate cellular activation by Mycobacterium tuberculosis. J Immunol 1999;163:3920-7.
61. Schwandner R, Dziarski R, Wesche H, Rothe M, Kirschning CJ. Peptidoglycan- and lipoteichoic acid-induced cell activation is mediated by toll-like receptor 2. J Biol Chem 1999;274:17406-9.
62. Yoshimura A, Lien E, Ingalls RR, Tuomanen E, Dziarski R, Golenbock D. Cutting edge: recognition of Gram-positive bacterial cell wall components by the innate immune system occurs via Toll-like receptor 2. J Immunol 1999;163:1-5.
63. Takeuchi O, Hoshino K, Kawai T, Sanjo H, Takada H, Ogawa T, et al. Differential roles of TLR2 and TLR4 in recognition of gram-negative and gram-positive bacterial cell wall components. Immunity 1999;11:443-51.
64. Lien E, Sellati TJ, Yoshimura A, Flo TH, Rawadi G, Finberg RW, et al. Toll-like receptor 2 functions as a pattern recognition receptor for diverse bacterial products. J Biol Chem 1999;274:33419-25.
65. Tapping RI, Tobias PS. Soluble CD14-mediated cellular responses to lipopolysaccharide. Chem Immunol 2000;74:108-21.
66. Poltorak A, Smirnova I, He X, Liu MY, Van Huffel C, McNally O, et al. Genetic and physical mapping of the Lps locus: identification of the toll-4 receptor as a candidate gene in the critical region. Blood Cells Mol Dis 1998;24:340-55.
67. Poltorak A, He X, Smirnova I, Liu MY, Huffel CV, Du X, et al. Defective LPS signaling in C3H/HeJ and C57BL/10ScCr mice: mutations in Tlr4 gene. Science 1998;282:2085-8.
68. Qureshi ST, Lariviere L, Leveque G, Clermont S, Moore KJ, Gros P, et al. Endotoxin-tolerant mice have mutations in Toll-like receptor 4 (Tlr4). J Exp Med 1999;189:615-25.
69. Hoshino K, Takeuchi O, Kawai T, Sanjo H, Ogawa T, Takeda Y, et al. Cutting edge: Toll-like receptor 4 (TLR4)-deficient mice are hyporesponsive to lipopolysaccharide: evidence for TLR4 as the Lps gene product. J Immunol 1999;162:3749-52.

70. Chow JC, Young DW, Golenbock DT, Christ WJ, Gusovsky F. Toll-like receptor-4 mediates lipopolysaccharide-induced signal transduction. J Biol Chem 1999;274:10689-92.
71. Akashi S, Ogata H, Kirikae F, Kirikae T, Kawasaki K, Nishijima M, et al. Regulatory roles for CD14 and phosphatidylinositol in the signaling via toll-like receptor 4-MD-2. Biochem Biophys Res Commun 2000;268:172-7.
72. Heine H, Kirschning CJ, Lien E, Monks BG, Rothe M, Golenbock DT. Cutting edge: cells that carry A null allele for toll-like receptor 2 are capable of responding to endotoxin. J Immunol 1999;162:6971-5.
73. Lien E, Means TK, Heine H, Yoshimura A, Kusumoto S, Fukase K, et al. Toll-like receptor 4 imparts ligand-specific recognition of bacterial lipopolysaccharide. J Clin Invest 2000;105:497-504.
74. Kawasaki K, Akashi S, Shimazu R, Yoshida T, Miyake K, Nishijima M. Mouse toll-like receptor 4.MD-2 complex mediates lipopolysaccharide- mimetic signal transduction by Taxol. J Biol Chem 2000;275:2251-4.
75. Tobias PS, Soldau K, Kline L, Lee JD, Kato K, Martin TP, et al. Cross-linking of lipopolysaccharide (LPS) to CD14 on THP-1 cells mediated by LPS-binding protein. J Immunol 1993;150:3011-21.
76. Poussin C, Foti M, Carpentier JL, Pugin J. CD14-dependent endotoxin internalization via a macropinocytic pathway. J Biol Chem 1998;273:20285-91.
77. Ding A, Thieblemont N, Zhu J, Jin F, Zhang J, Wright SD. Secretory leukocyte protease inhibitor interferes with uptake of lipopolysaccharide by macrophages. Infect Immun 1999;67:4485-4489.
78. Gregory CD. CD14-dependent clearance of apoptotic cells: relevance to the immune system. Curr Opin Immunol 2000;12:27-34.
79. Schiff DE, Kline L, Soldau K, Lee JD, Pugin J, Tobias PS, et al. Phagocytosis of gram-negative bacteria by a unique CD14-dependent mechanism. J Leukoc Biol 1997;62:786-94.
80. Underhill DM, Ozinsky A, Hajjar AM, Stevens A, Wilson CB, Bassetti M, et al. The Toll-like receptor 2 is recruited to macrophage phagosomes and discriminates between pathogens. Nature 1999;401:811-5.
81. Frantz S, Kobzik L, Kim YD, Fukazawa R, Medzhitov R, Lee RT, et al. Toll4 (TLR4) expression in cardiac myocytes in normal and failing myocardium. J Clin Invest 1999;104:271-80.
82. Ohashi K, Burkart V, Flohe S, Kolb H. Cutting edge: heat shock protein 60 is a putative endogenous ligand of the toll-like receptor-4 complex. J Immunol 2000;164:558-61.
83. Nomura F, Akashi S, Sakao Y, Sato S, Kawai T, Matsumoto M, et al. Cutting edge: endotoxin tolerance in mouse peritoneal macrophages correlates with down-regulation of surface toll-like receptor 4 expression. J Immunol 2000;164:3476-9.
84. Staege H, Schaffner A, Schneemann M. Human toll-like receptors 2 and 4 are targets for deactivation of mononuclear phagocytes by interleukin-4. Immunol Lett 2000;71:1-3.
85. Miura Y, Shimazu R, Miyake K, Akashi S, Ogata H, Yamashita Y, et al. RP105 is associated with MD-1 and transmits an activation signal in human B cells. Blood 1998;92:2815-22.
86. Miyake K, Shimazu R, Kondo J, Niki T, Akashi S, Ogata H, et al. Mouse MD-1, a molecule that is physically associated with RP105 and positively regulates its expression. J Immunol 1998;161:1348-53.

87. Shimazu R, Akashi S, Ogata H, Nagai Y, Fukudome K, Miyake K, et al. MD-2, a molecule that confers lipopolysaccharide responsiveness on Toll- like receptor 4. J Exp Med 1999;189:1777-82.
88. Underhill DM, Ozinsky A, Smith KD, Aderem A. Toll-like receptor-2 mediates mycobacteria-induced proinflammatory signaling in macrophages. Proc Natl Acad Sci U S A 1999;96:14459-63.
89. Takeuchi O, Takeda K, Hoshino K, Adachi O, Ogawa T, Akira S. Cellular responses to bacterial cell wall components are mediated through MyD88-dependent signaling cascades. Int Immunol 2000;12:113-7.
90. Takeuchi O, Kaufmann A, Grote K, Kawai T, Hoshino K, Morr M, et al. Cutting edge: preferentially the R-stereoisomer of the mycoplasmal lipopeptide macrophage-activating lipopeptide-2 activates immune cells through a toll-like receptor 2- and MyD88-dependent signaling pathway. J Immunol 2000;164:554-7.
91. Taylor MJ, Cross HF, Bilo K. Inflammatory responses induced by the filarial nematode brugia malayi are mediated by lipopolysaccharide-like activity from endosymbiotic wolbachia bacteria. J Exp Med 2000;191:1429-36.
92. Chan VW, Mecklenbrauker I, Su I, Texido G, Leitges M, Carsetti R, et al. The molecular mechanism of B cell activation by toll-like receptor protein RP-105. J Exp Med 1998;188:93-101.
93. Medzhitov R, Preston-Hurlburt P, Kopp E, Stadlen A, Chen C, Ghosh S, et al. MyD88 is an adaptor protein in the hToll/IL-1 receptor family signaling pathways. Mol Cell 1998;2:253-8.
94. Muzio M, Ni J, Feng P, Dixit VM. IRAK (Pelle) family member IRAK-2 and MyD88 as proximal mediators of IL- 1 signaling. Science 1997;278:1612-5.
95. Wesche H, Henzel WJ, Shillinglaw W, Li S, Cao Z. MyD88: an adapter that recruits IRAK to the IL-1 receptor complex. Immunity 1997;7:837-47.
96. Burns K, Martinon F, Esslinger C, Pahl H, Schneider P, Bodmer JL, et al. MyD88, an adapter protein involved in interleukin-1 signaling. J Biol Chem 1998;273:12203-9.
97. Swantek JL, Tsen MF, Cobb MH, Thomas JA. IL-1 receptor-associated kinase modulates host responsiveness to endotoxin. J Immunol 2000;164:4301-6.
98. Muzio M, Natoli G, Saccani S, Levrero M, Mantovani A. The human toll signaling pathway: divergence of nuclear factor kappaB and JNK/SAPK activation upstream of tumor necrosis factor receptor- associated factor 6 (TRAF6). J Exp Med 1998;187:2097-101.
99. Irie T, Muta T, Takeshige K. TAK1 mediates an activation signal from toll-like receptor(s) to nuclear factor-kappaB in lipopolysaccharide-stimulated macrophages. FEBS Lett 2000;467:160-4.
100. Kawai T, Adachi O, Ogawa T, Takeda K, Akira S. Unresponsiveness of MyD88-deficient mice to endotoxin. Immunity 1999;11:115-22.
101. Kuhns DB, Long Priel DA, Gallin JI. Endotoxin and IL-1 hyporesponsiveness in a patient with recurrent bacterial infections. J Immunol 1997;158:3959-3964.

Chapter 4

MACROPHAGE MIGRATION INHIBITORY FACTOR (MIF): A PRO-INFLAMMATORY MEDIATOR OF SEPSIS

Christian Martin, Ph.D., Thierry Roger, Ph.D., Thierry Calandra, M.D.,Ph.D.
Division of Infectious Diseases, Department of Internal Medicine, Centre Hospitalier Universitaire Vaudois, CH-1011 Lausanne, Switzerland

Introduction

Over the last ten years, the protein known as macrophage migration inhibitory factor (MIF) has emerged to be a central cytokine of the innate immune system and was found to play an important part in the control of inflammatory responses. MIF is considered to be one of the first cytokine activities described. Investigations of the mechanisms of delayed-type hypersensitivity reactions conducted in the late 1960s have led to the recognition of an activity that inhibited the random migration of guinea pig peritoneal exudate cells. In 1966, Bloom and David associated this macrophage migration inhibitory activity to a soluble, non-dialyzable factor released by sensitized lymphocytes (1,2). These reports stimulated the curiosity of immunologists as MIF was one of the first lymphokines to be described. Over the next 20 years, MIF was found to enhance a broad-spectrum of macrophage functions, including adherence, phagocytosis, spreading, and tumoricidal activity (reviewed in reference 3). The biological activities ascribed to MIF remained uncertain as cytokines such IFNγ and IL-4 also were observed to inhibit macrophage migration. The cloning of a human MIF cDNA in 1989 was a milestone in the investigations of the biochemical and biological properties of MIF (4). However, initial studies were performed with unpurified recombinant MIF protein that was later found to contain a mitogenic contaminant.

In the early 1990s, MIF was re-discovered as a pituitary peptide during investigations of factors that may serve to control inflammatory responses induced by sepsis. LPS-stimulated AtT-20 anterior pituitary cells were found to release copious amounts of a 12.5-kDa protein (5). N-terminal sequencing of the protein revealed that this protein was the mouse homologue of human MIF and shared 90% identity with human MIF. Cloning and sequencing of an AtT-20 MIF cDNA confirmed these results. Additional experiments indicated that MIF was secreted from the pituitary gland and from the adrenal cortex in a hormone-like fashion after LPS stimulation (6,7). These initial observations provided the impetus to clone the mouse and human *Mif* genes, to express recombinant proteins and produce antibodies to study the biological activities of MIF.

In recent years, several comprehensive reviews of the biochemical and biological properties of MIF have been published (3,8,9). The objective of the present review is to focus on the role played by MIF in host responses against infection.

MIF GENE AND GENE REGULATION

Cloning and Characterization

The human and mouse *Mif* genes have been cloned (10,11). The mouse *Mif* gene has been mapped to chromosome 10 and lies between the Bcr and S100b loci (11,12). At least nine *Mif* pseudogenes have been identified in the mouse genome (12,13). A mouse *Mif* gene isolated from the liver was shown to be composed of three exons and two short introns of 201 and 145 nucleotides (11). The position of mouse *Mif* gene on chromosome 10 is coincident with several recessive mutations, including the gray lethal (gl), mocha (mh), and grizzled (gr) (11). However, there is no indication that mutations of the *Mif* gene result in any known mouse defect or disease. In fact, MIF knockout mice exhibit a normal phenotype and were reported to be healthy (14). In contrast to mouse *Mif*, human *Mif* was reported to exist as a single functional gene without pseudogenes (10). It was mapped to a region of chromosome 22 (22q11.2) known to be in syntenic conservation with a section of mouse chromosome 10 containing the *Mif* gene (15). The genomic structure of human *Mif* is analogous to mouse *Mif* and contains three exons spanning less than 1 kb that are separated by small introns (189 and 95 bp). Predicted coding sequence of the *Mif* gene was identical to sequences of the *Mif* cDNA of the human eye lens (16) and the Jurkat human

T-cell line (17). A single MIF mRNA band of approximately 0.8 kb was found in all human tissues examined by Northern blotting. Like in the mouse, many human organs, including the kidney, brain and liver, expressed high MIF mRNA levels at baseline. The mouse and human *Mif* genes exhibit a high degree of homology within each exon (70.4%, 86.4% and 67.5% for exons 1, 2 and 3, respectively). Except for D-dopachrome tautomerase that shares about 30% homology with *Mif*, no noteworthy homology have been identified between *Mif* and any other DNA sequences (18).

Promoter Elements

Analysis of the 5'-regulatory region of the mouse *Mif* gene revealed the presence of several consensus sequences for transcription factors. The promoter region comprises sequence motifs implicated in the basal expression of the proto-oncogene *c-fos*, an Sp-1 site, a c-AMP responsive element (CRE), an AP-2 site, and an alleged negative glucocorticoid responsive element (nGRE) (11). All have been identified within 1 kb of the RNA transcription start, except for a cytokine-1 (CK-1) and a nuclear factor-κB (NF-κB) site located further upstream on the minus DNA strand. Functional studies of the mouse MIF promoter showed that CRE binding protein (CREB) mediated corticotrophin releasing factor (CRF)-induced *Mif* gene transcription in pituitary cells (19). Sequence analyses of the 5' region flanking the human MIF gene also revealed the presence of CRE and multiple Sp-1 sites (10).

STRUCTURE OF THE MIF PROTEIN

Mouse and human MIF display 90% identity of their amino acid sequences. Overall, the MIF proteins exhibit more than 80% homology across the species examined (mouse, rat, gerbil, chicken, calf, and human) and comprise an invariant proline residue at the N-terminus. For example, mouse and rat MIF differ only by one amino acid residue. MIF is identical to a protein known as glycosylation-inhibiting factor (GIF). GIF has been shown to suppress IgE synthesis and be associated with antigen-specific suppressor activity (20). Homologues of the MIF protein have been reported in *Caenorhabditis elegans*, *Arabidopsis thaliana* and in filarial parasites (*Wuchereria bancrofti*, *Brugia malayi* and *Onchocerca volvulus*). MIF shares a 33% amino acid sequence homology with D-dopachrome tautomerase (21). No significant sequence homology have been found between MIF and other cytokines, indicating that it does not belong to any cytokine superfamily. MIF and D-dopachrome tautomerase may be two members of a new protein superfamily. Like IL-1, basic FGF, and a secreted form of cyclophilin, MIF lack a classical N-terminal leader sequence and is thus released from cells by a nonconventional protein secretion pathway. Two potential N-glycosylation sites have been identified at positions 75 and 110, but structural analysis of native MIF by mass spectrometry or enzymatic studies have ruled out any detectable, post-translational - glycosylation.

Crystal Structure

The crystal structure of human and rat MIF have been solved (22,23). It has revealed that MIF is a trimer with dimensions of 35 x 50 x 50 Å. MIF monomer consists of two antiparallel α-helices and six β-strands. The secondary and tertiary structure of MIF display a pseudo-twofold symmetry with a βαβββαββ sequence. The pseudo-twofold symmetry axis is perpendicular to the β-sheet. The β1, β2, and β4 sheets form the inner part of the trimer and wrap around so that the trimer has the form of a barrel with a solvent-accessible channel. Despite no sequence homology, significant three-dimensional structural homology have been found between MIF and two bacterial isomerases, 4-oxalocrotonate tautomerase (4-OT) and 5-carboxymethyl-2-hydroxymuconate isomerase (CHMI) (24). Readers interested in a more detailed discussion of the three-dimensional structure of MIF should refer to an excellent review article on this topic (9).

Enzymatic Activity

Purified recombinant MIF protein was found recently to exhibit a tautomerase activity catalyzing the conversion of the melanogenic substrate 2-carboxy-2,3-dihydroindole-5,6-quinone (dopachrome) into 5,6-dihydroxyindole-2-carboxylic acid (DHICA) (25,26). These observations have suggested the intriguing possibility that MIF may exert some of its biological effects by catalyzing an enzymatic reaction. However, *D*-dopachrome is not a naturally-occurring product and natural MIF substrates thus remain to be identified. Interestingly, the fact that MIF displays an isomerization activity bears some resemblance with the situation described for cyclophilin. Cyclophilin, the target for the immunosuppressant drug cyclosporin A, has been shown to act intracellularly as a peptidyl-prolyl *cis-trans* isomerase, and very much like MIF was found to be released from cells in response to pro-inflammatory stimuli. The catalytic activity of MIF was linked to the N-terminal proline of the protein as deletion or replacement of this amino acid residue abolished the enzymatic activity (27). Other enzymatic properties have been ascribed to MIF. These include the enolization of phenylpyruvate and the ketonization of p-hydroxyphenylpyruvate (26). However, the physiological significance of the enzymatic activity linked to MIF remains unclear. Substitution of the N-terminal proline by a serine abrogated the tautomerization activity of MIF, but not its glucocorticoid counter-regulatory activity (27). Consistent with these initial observations, it was recently observed that MIF mutants in which the N-terminal proline was replaced either with a serine or with a phenylalanine exhibited reduced or no phenylpyruvate tautomerase activity, yet they remain capable of inhibiting monocyte chemotaxis and random migration (28). These data strongly suggest that the immunological or migration inhibiting properties of MIF are not mediated by an enzymatic activity. Chromosomal mapping of the *Mif* and dopachrome tautomerase genes have shown that they are in close proximity. It is therefore conceivable that both genes arose by duplication of a common ancestral gene and have evolved to exhibit different functions. MIF was reported to exert a thiol-protein oxidoreductase activity (29). Work is in progress to elucidate the biological relevance of this finding.

CELLULAR SOURCES OF MIF WITHIN THE IMMUNE SYSTEM

As shown in Table 1, the MIF protein displays a wide tissue distribution. We will focus our attention on the cellular sources of MIF within the immune system as the objective of the present article is to review the role played by MIF in host responses against infection.

Monocytes and Macrophages

Originally, T cells were thought to be the main cellular source of MIF and macrophages considered to be the main cellular target of MIF released by T-cells. However, in 1994 cells of the monocyte/macrophage lineage were identified to be an abundant source of MIF (6). Unlike other cytokines, high baseline levels of MIF mRNA and MIF protein were detected in resting macrophages. Macrophages release MIF when stimulated with microbial products [LPS, toxic shock syndrome toxin-1 (TSST-1), streptococcal pyrogenic exotoxin A (SPEA) and malaria pigment], bacteria (Gram-negative and Gram-positive, *M. tuberculosis*) and cytokines (TNFα and IFNγ) (6,30-32) (Oddo M et al., unpublished). Of note, macrophage MIF secretion is induced by very low concentrations of LPS, TSST-1 or SPEA. Production of MIF by macrophages follows a classical bell-shaped curve that may protect the host from the detrimental effect of excessive concentrations of this powerful pro-inflammatory cytokine. MIF induces TNFα secretion by macrophages and synergizes with IFNγ to augment nitric

Table 1. Tissue Distribution and Cellular Sources of MIF

Immune system:
Monocytes/macrophages, T cells, B cells
Eosinophils, mast cells, basophils
Neutrophils
Spleen (white pulp, red pulp)
Endocrine system:
Pituitary gland (corticotrophic cells)
Adrenal cortex (zona glomerulosa, zona fasciculata)
Pancreas (β cells of the islet)
Brain:
Cortex (neurons), hypothalamus, cerebellum (neurons), hippocampus, pons, glial cells, ependyma
Kidney:
Epithelial cells (proximal tubules, collecting ducts, glomeruli Bowman's capsule), mesangial cells
Lung:
Alveolar macrophages, epithelial cells (bronchi)
Liver:
Kuppfer cells, hepatocytes, endothelium (central venules)
Gastrointestinal tract:
Epithelial cells (esophagus, stomach, small and large intestines)
Neurons (myenteric and submucosal plexi)
Skin:
Keratinocytes, sebaceous gland, hair follicle (outer root sheet) endothelial cells, fibroblasts
Eye:
Lens, epithelial cells (cornea, iris, ciliary body), endothelial cells, retina (epithelium, Müller cells, astrocytes)
Testis:
Leydig cells
Prostate:
Epithelial cells
Ovary:
Granulosa cells of follicles
Bone:
Osteoblasts
Fat tissue:
Adipocytes
Vasculature:
Endothelial cells

oxide production, and thus works in concert with these two cytokines to intensify pro-inflammatory responses of macrophages (6,17). Unexpectedly, glucocorticoid hormones were found to induce, rather than to inhibit MIF secretion (33). As observed with bacterial toxins, glucocorticoid-induced macrophage MIF production also showed a bell-shaped dose response curve. Peak MIF release occurred at concentrations of dexamethasone in the range of 10^{-12}-10^{-14} M. Similar results were obtained when macrophages were stimulated with cortisol. The implication of the paradoxical observation that glucocorticoids stimulate the release of a pro-inflammatory cytokine is discussed below.

T Cells

Even though MIF was discovered originally as a factor released by lymphocytes, relatively little is known about the effect of MIF on either T cells or B cells, presumably because the macrophage was thought to be the main cellular target of MIF. As observed for macrophages, pre-formed MIF protein was detected in resting T cells (34). T cells purified from mouse spleen or human peripheral blood expressed MIF mRNA and MIF protein, which is released after stimulation with mitogen, anti-CD3 antibody, and specific antigen (34). MIF was found to be produced predominantly by the T_H2 subset of helper T cells. Subsequent experiments showed that the staphylococcal superantigen TSST-1 was a very powerful inducer of MIF secretion from mouse splenocytes (30). MIF secretion was induced by concentrations of TSST-1 that were much lower than those required to trigger IL-2 or IFNγ secretion (10 pg/ml versus 1 ng/ml). Subsequent studies established that MIF contributes to T cell activation *in vivo*. Anti-MIF antibodies inhibited T cell proliferation and IL-2 production *in vitro* (34). In agreement with the observation that MIF is released by T_H2 lymphocytes, anti-MIF antibody also suppressed antigen-driven T cell activation and antibody production *in vivo*. Moreover, pretreatment of mice with neutralizing anti-MIF antibody prior to injection of the superantigenic staphylococcal exotoxin TSST-1 prevented spleen enlargement and reduced by half the proliferation of splenocytes measured *ex vivo* 72 hr after TSST-1 challenge (30). These results therefore indicate that MIF exerts autocrine effects on T cells and contributes to the mitogenic response of lymphocytes after activation with staphylococcal exotoxins, tetanus toxoid or anti-CD3 antibodies. Glucocorticoids also induced MIF secretion by T cells in a concentration-dependent manner (34). Work is in progress to characterize the role played by MIF in T-cell mediated immunity.

B Cells

Previous studies have suggested a role for MIF in activation of B cells. Anti-MIF antibody were shown to inhibit antibody production by B cells (34). More recently, MIF protein was reported to be released in copious amounts by an Epstein-Barr virus-transformed human B-cell line (35). Interestingly, MIF was observed to bind to HLA-DRB1*0405 via the amino acid sequence Y36IAV39, confirming a part for MIF in B cell activation. MIF protein was also detected in the WEHI 231 B-cell line (36). In contrast to wild-type WEHI 231 B-cells or cells transfected with a control vector, cells transfected with a MIF antisense plasmid (WaM2), that decreased the levels of endogenous MIF protein, displayed reduced growth arrest and apoptosis after crosslinking of IgM. This was associated with a reduced proportion of cells in G1 phase and an increased proportion of cells in S phase. These experiments therefore suggest a role for MIF in the control of cell cycle progression and apoptosis in B cells.

Neutrophils

Together with complement, neutrophils are the first line of host defenses against invading micro-organisms and as such are a critical element of the innate immune system. MIF protein is expressed in neutrophils (37). However, it is expressed in much lower quantities than in macrophages or T cells, as shown by the fact that initial Western blotting analysis of the MIF content of human neutrophils with anti-mouse MIF antibodies yielded negative results, while macrophages and T cells showed strongly positive signals (6). Pretreatment of neutrophils with recombinant MIF resulted in an augmentation of superoxide production after stimulation with FMLP (37), suggesting that MIF might exert a priming effect on neutrophils. Recombinant MIF was found to augment chemoattractant-induced luminol- and lucigenin-amplified neutrophil chemiluminescence, but inhibited phorbol myristate acetate (PMA) –induced neutrophil luminol-amplified chemiluminescence. (M. Markert and T. Calandra, unpublished). Administration of anti-MIF antibody to rats decreased LPS-induced influx of neutrophils into the lungs and reduced the myeloperoxidase activity in lung tissue (38). Compared to heterozygous or wild-type mice, MIF knockout mice had lower neutrophils counts in the BAL after the instillation of *Pseudomonas aeruginosa* into the trachea and enhanced clearance of the bacteria (14).

Eosinophils, Mast Cells and Basophils

Allergic reactions often follow a bimodal course with an early and a late phase. Mast cells and basophils play an important role in the early phase, while eosinophils are the main cellular component of the late phase. Given the important contribution of MIF in inflammatory responses and the role played by eosinophils, mast cells and basophils in the pathogenesis of allergic diseases, researchers measured the concentrations of MIF in the broncho-alveolar lavage (BAL) of asthmatic patients and looked for the cellular sources of MIF. As anticipated, elevated concentrations of MIF were detected in the BAL of these patients (39). Like monocytes, macrophages, T cells and B cells, unstimulated eosinophils were described to also be an abundant cellular source of MIF (39). Stimulation of human eosinophils with C5a, IL-5 and phorbol myristate acetate (PMA) induced an immediate release of MIF protein. The finding of elevated concentrations of MIF in the BAL of asthmatic patients may have potential therapeutic implications. Indeed, anti-MIF strategy might help to control excessive airway inflammation, which is a key feature of allergic pulmonary reactions. Furthermore, MIF mRNA and protein were identified in mast cells isolated from the rat peritoneum (40). The human HMC-1 immature mast cell line and in the KU812 basophil cell line constitutively express and secrete high amounts of MIF (40).

Natural Killer Cells

Together with monocytes, macrophages and neutrophils, natural killer (NK) cells contribute to innate immune responses. During the course of studies that examined the mechanisms sustaining immune privilege in the anterior chamber of the rabbit eye, a factor sharing more than 90% homology with residues 95-108 of human MIF was shown to inhibit the NK-mediated lysis of corneal endothelial cells (41). Of note, recombinant mouse MIF inhibited NK activity and neutralizing anti-MIF restored it. Yet, MIF was not directly toxic to NK cells, but exerted its effects by interfering with the release of cytolytic perforin granules from NK cells. Interestingly, MIF did not affect perforin release by allospecific cytotoxic T lymphocytes (CTL) and did not inhibit CTL-mediated cytolysis of allogeneic target cells. It is unclear whether NK cells express MIF protein. Yet, the eye lens, the iris and the cornea and tissue macrophages are well-known sources of MIF that may act locally on NK cells (16,42).

BIOLOGICAL ACTIVITIES OF MIF

The main properties and biological activities of MIF are reported in Table 2.

Table 2. Properties and Biological Activities of MIF

Innate Immunity and Inflammation	Inhibition of macrophage migration Pituitary peptide, macrophage and T cell cytokine secreted in response to pro- and anti-inflammatory stimuli (endotoxins;exotoxins: TSST-1, SPEA; PPD; malaria pigment; cytokines: TNFα, IFNγ ; glucocorticoids) Activation of macrophages (promotes cytokine and NO production, phagocytosis of particles and killing of micro-organisms) Critical mediator of septic shock (endotoxemia, TSST-1-induced shock, *E. coli* peritonitis, cecal ligation and puncture peritonitis) Counter-regulator of the anti-inflammatory effects of glucocorticoids (macrophages) Involved in the pathogenesis of glomerulonephritis and arthritis Involved in the pathophysiology of malaria anemia
Acquired immunity	Required for antigen-dependent T cell proliferation, antibody production by B cells and delayed-type hypersensitivity reaction Counter-regulator of the immunosuppressive effects of glucocorticoids (T cells)
Glucose metabolism	Promotes insulin release from cells of the islet of Langerhans Regulates glycolysis by inducing expression of 6-phosphofructo-2-kinase/fructose-2,6-bisphophatase (PFK-2)
Angiogenesis	Promotes proliferation of endothelial cells
Cell growth	Mitogen for fibroblasts Promotes proliferation of tumor cells
Enzymatic activity	Tautomerase activity Oxidoreductase activity

MIF as a Mediator of Sepsis

The fact that MIF was rediscovered in the early 1990s as a pituitary and macrophage mediator induced by microbial products (LPS, TSST-1, SPEA) and cytokines (TNFα and IFNγ) suggested a role for MIF in host defenses against infection (5,6,30). Subsequent studies have confirmed a critical part for MIF in innate immunity. Immunohistochemistry, Western blotting and *in situ* hybridization analyses have revealed that MIF is also expressed constitutively in several cell types of numerous organs, including lung, liver, spleen, kidney, pituitary gland, adrenal gland and skin (6,7). Administration of LPS in the rat was accompanied within 6 hours by a release of pre-formed MIF protein from nearly all tissues examined. This was followed by a strong induction of MIF mRNA resulting in restoration of supranormal levels of intracellular MIF at 24 hours (7). Similar to TNFα and IL-1, MIF is a critical mediator of experimental endotoxemia, even though it does not induce hypotension when injected intravenously in rodents. Recombinant MIF aggravates lethal endotoxemia when co-injected with LPS into mice. On the contrary, neutralizing anti-MIF antibodies fully protect mice from endotoxic shock (5). Increased survival was associated with a 50% reduction of the circulating levels of TNFα (Bernhagen et al., unpublished). Confirming the initial results obtained with anti-MIF antibodies, mice with deletion of the MIF gene were reported to be resistant to endotoxic shock (14). Of note, serum levels of TNFα, but not of IL-6 or IL-10, were lower in MIF knockout mice than in wild-type endotoxemic mice.

MIF also is implicated in the immune responses induced by staphylococcal and streptococcal exotoxins. Low concentrations of TSST-1 and SPEA were found to induce the release of MIF from macrophages and anti-MIF antibodies prevented death in a mouse model of toxic shock syndrome caused by the staphylococcal exotoxin TSST-1 (30). Moreover, anti-MIF antibodies also decreased lymphocyte proliferation stimulated by the superantigenic TSST-1. MIF knockout mice also were resistant to shock induced by staphylococcal enterotoxin B in galactosamine-sensitized mice (14). Overall these studies showed that Gram-negative endotoxins and Gram-positive exotoxins are very potent inducers of MIF secretion by immune cells and established an important role for MIF in the pathogenesis of toxic shock syndromes.

To assess the role of MIF in the pathogenesis of septic shock caused by live bacteria, experiments were performed in two models of bacterial peritonitis that mimic one of the most frequent causes of septic shock in humans (31). Infection was elicited either by an intraperitoneal injection of *E. coli* or by cecal ligation and puncture (CLP). Development of bacterial peritonitis increased the concentrations of MIF in the peritoneum and in the blood. Anti-MIF antibody protected mice from lethal peritonitis induced by CLP and by *E. coli*, even when treatment was started as late as 8 hours after the onset of CLP (Figures 1 and 2) (31). Noteworthy, anti-MIF treatment also protected TNF knockout mice, which are exquisitely sensitive to CLP due to the inability to mount an immune response in the absence of this pivotal pro-inflammatory cytokine. The latter finding provided a direct evidence for an intrinsic contribution of MIF to the pathogenesis of sepsis. As was observed in experimental endotoxemia, anti-MIF therapy reduced plasma levels of TNFα, and to a lesser extent of IL-6, of mice with *E. coli* peritonitis. However, TNFα is probably not the main target of MIF-mediated effects in sepsis as treatment with anti-MIF antibody protected TNFα knockout mice from death. Survival advantage achieved with neutralization of MIF activity was associated with lower blood counts of *E. coli*. However, there was no evidence of a direct cause and effect relationship between anti-MIF therapy and bacterial counts. rMIF did not promote the growth of *E. coli in vitro*. Moreover, in contrast to the results obtained with anti-TNF agents, anti-MIF therapy did not increase mortality in mice challenged with an low inoculum of *E. coli* (31). Compared to wild-type mice, MIF knockout mice have been shown to clear *Pseudomonas aeruginosa* instilled into the trachea better than wild-type mice and had lower neutrophil counts in their broncho-alveolar fluid. Taken together, these results suggest that bacterial clearance is an early marker of improved outcome rather than a primary target of anti-MIF-mediated effects. Furthermore, mice treated with anti-MIF IgG had similar serum levels of corticosterone than those treated with control IgG, as measured 12 hours after the onset of *E. coli* peritonitis (T. Calandra, unpublished). Thus, neutralization of MIF activity did not increase the circulating levels of glucocorticoids, suggesting that the protective effects of MIF were not mediated by an augmentation of endogenous glucocorticoid hormones. What could then be the mechanism by which MIF plays a detrimental role in septic shock? MIF was shown recently to stimulate cytosolic phospholipase A_2 activity and arachidonic acid release by fibroblasts (43). Activation of the arachidonic acid-prostaglandins-leukotrienes pathway might be an important component of MIF-mediated effect in sepsis. Experiments carried out with macrophages expressing an antisense MIF cDNA plasmid have revealed an important role for MIF in LPS signaling (T. Roger, manuscript in preparation). On the other hand, lethality of peritonitis was increased when mice were co-injected with rMIF and *E. coli*, thus supporting the concept that elevated tissue or blood levels of MIF are harmful. In fact, high levels of MIF were detected in the plasma of patients with severe sepsis or septic shock caused by Gram-negative or by Gram-positive bacteria (31). Median concentrations of MIF were 12.2 ng/ml (range: 6.2 to 141.8 ng/ml) and 17.8 ng/ml (range: 6.6 to 154.4 ng/ml) in patients with severe sepsis and septic shock, respectively, compared with 3 ng/ml (range: 1.9-5.4 ng/ml) in healthy controls (P values were 0.001 and 0.0004 for controls versus patients with severe sepsis or septic shock, respectively, and 0.3 for patients with severe sepsis versus septic shock) (Figure 3).

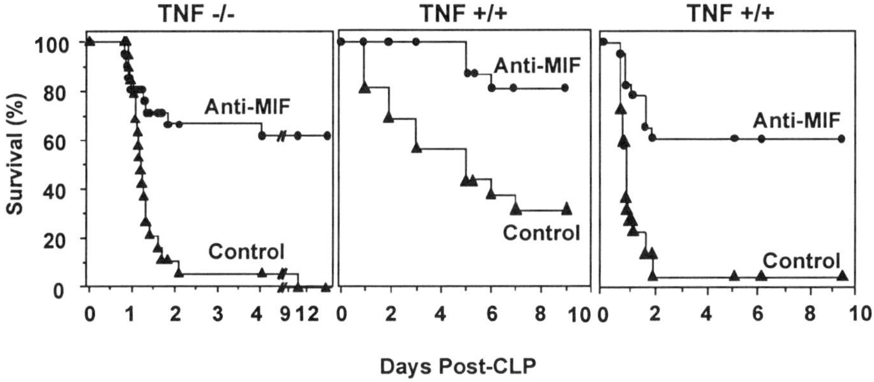

Figure 1. Anti-MIF monoclonal antibodies (mAb) protect TNF knockout (TNF -/-) and wild-type (TNF +/+) mice from septic shock induced by cecal ligation and puncture. Left panel : Survival : Anti-MIF mAb : 62% , control antibody : 0%, P=0.00002. Middle panel : Anti-MIF mAb was given at the time of surgery (t=0h), survival : Anti-MIF mAb : 81%, control antibody : 31% , P=0.01. Right panel : Anti-MIF mAb was given 4.5 h after surgery, survival : Anti-MIF mAb 61%, control antibody : 5%, P=0.00008. Adapted from reference #31 with permission.

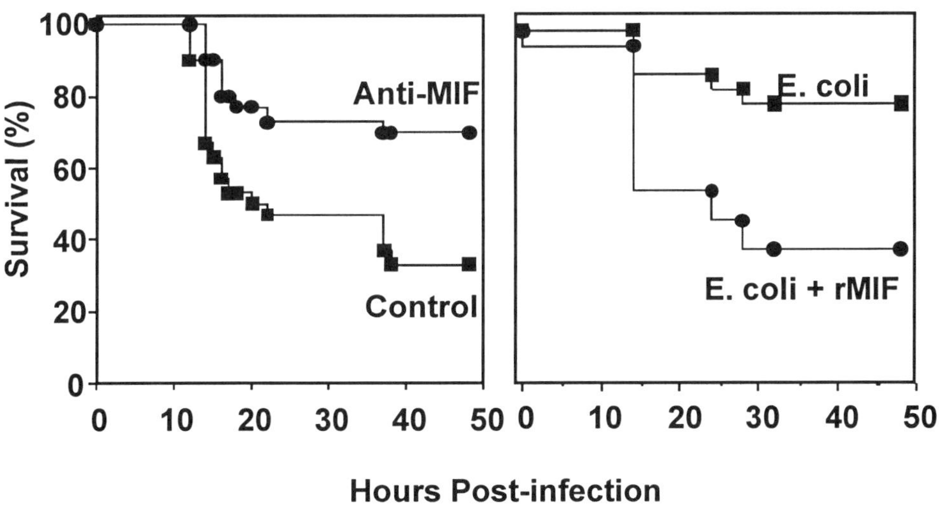

Figure 2. Anti-MIF IgG protects against lethal *E. coli* peritonitis (left panel). Survival : anti-MIF IgG : 70%, control antibody : 33%, P=0.009. MIF potentiates lethality of *E. coli* peritonitis (right panel). Mortality : *E. coli* alone: 21%, *E. coli* + rMIF : 62 %, P=0.008. Adapted from reference #31 with permission.

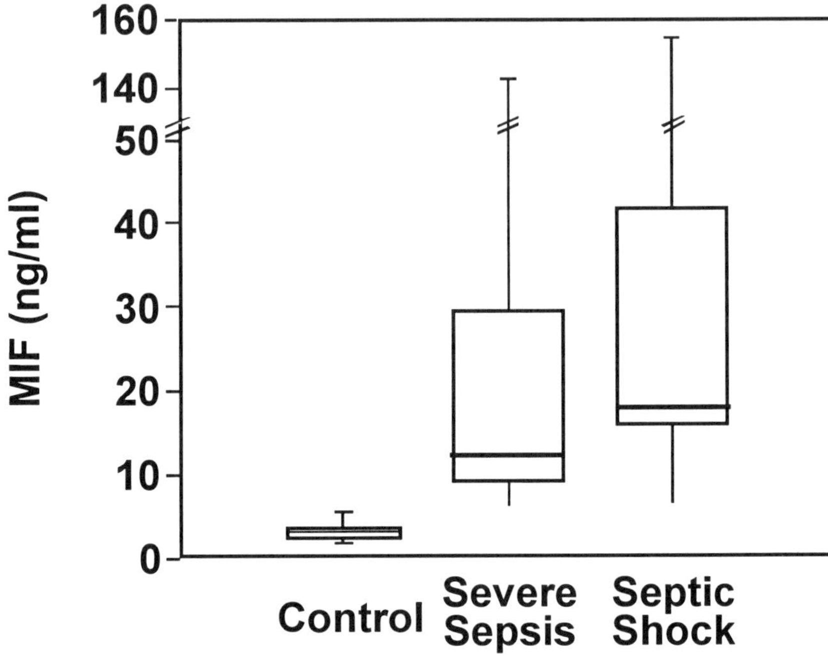

Figure 3. Boxplots of the plasma concentrations of MIF of healthy individuals (controls) (n=6) and of patients with either severe sepsis (n=7) or septic shock (n=9). The bottom, median and top lines of the box mark the 25th, 50th and 75th percentiles, respectively. The vertical line shows the range of values comprised between the 5th and 95th percentiles. Reproduced from reference #31 with permission.

In addition to septic shock, MIF was shown to be involved in the pathophysiology of malaria and leishmaniasis. Ingestion of erythrocytes infected with *Plasmadia chabaudi* or malarial pigment (hemozoin) by macrophages stimulated the release of MIF (32). Interestingly, MIF was found to inhibit erythroid, multipotential, and granulocyte-macrophage progenitor-derived colony formation, suggesting that MIF could be implicated in the pathophysiology of malaria anemia. MIF mRNA and protein have been detected in the lymph nodes of mice infected with *Leishmania major* (44). Consistent with the macrophage activating properties of MIF, recombinant MIF increased the killing of *Leishmania major* by macrophages in a TNFα- and nitric oxide-dependent fashion. Furthermore, MIF delivered orally by a *Salmonella* strain engineered to express cytokines reduced the severity of infection in an experimental

Leishmania model (45). Taken together these studies define a critical role for MIF in the pathogenesis of septic shock and in innate immune responses induced by a wide range of microorganisms. They also identify MIF as a potential novel target for therapeutic intervention in patients with severe sepsis and possibly also with other infectious diseases.

Pathophysiological Role in Other Inflammatory Diseases

Elevated concentrations of MIF were detected in alveolar airspaces of patients with the adult respiratory distress syndrome (ARDS) (46). Recombinant MIF was found to augment IL-8 and TNFα secretion by alveolar cells of ARDS patients, whereas incubation of cells in the presence of anti-MIF antibodies decreased the production of both cytokines. Expression of MIF is up-regulated in patients with rheumatoid arthritis (RA). MIF mRNA and protein were detected in the synovium of patients with RA. Infiltrating mononuclear cells (T cells and macrophages) and fibroblast-like synoviocytes were identified to be the primary sources of MIF (47,48). Synovial fluid levels of MIF were higher in patients with RA than in patients with osteoarthritis (49). Stimulation of synoviocytes with pro-inflammatory cytokines (IL-1β, TNFα and IFNγ) did not augment MIF production (48). Depending upon the dose, dexamethasone exerted either stimulatory (10^{-10}-10^{-12}M) or inhibitory (10^{-7}M) effect on synoviocyte MIF expression (48). Patients with atopic dermatitis have been reported to have increased expression of MIF in keratinocytes and high circulating concentrations of MIF (50). Anti-MIF antibodies also reduced inflammation in experimental models of glomerulonephritis, and allograft rejection, confirming a role for MIF in the regulation of inflammatory responses.

MIF – Glucocorticoids Interactions

Inflammation is an essential component of host defenses against infectious agents. The cytokines released by leukocytes play a pivotal role in innate and acquired immune responses and act to coordinate the cellular and humoral responses that contribute to eradicate the infection or wall-off the invasive micro-organism. Because it is an essential feature of host defenses against infection, inflammatory responses need to be kept under tight control. On one hand, overwhelming inflammatory reactions are detrimental to the host and may even be lethal as seen in septic shock. On the other hand, the lack of inflammatory response typically encountered in immunocompromised patients may also be harmful by promoting life-threatening infections. The release of glucocorticoid hormones is a central feature of the physiological stress response induced by inflammation and infection. Glucocorticoids are potent anti-inflammatory and immunosuppressive agents and act as a sentinel to keep inflammatory responses in check. To control the development of the immune response, the host needs to balance the opposing effects of immunostimulatory and immunosuppressive molecules. By analogy with other physiological systems, it is reasonable to postulate that counter-regulatory systems should also exist within the immune system to maintain the equilibrium between pro-inflammatory and anti-inflammatory stimuli.

Recent data have suggested that MIF and glucocorticoids may function as a physiological counter-regulatory dyad to control host inflammatory and immune responses. As discussed above, MIF is produced by many cells of the immune system, including macrophages and the T lymphocytes (6,34). MIF is also stored in copious amounts in the pituitary gland and in the adrenal cortex, and is released in the systemic circulation during stress and infection (5,7,51). MIF exerts important functions within both the innate and acquired immune system. MIF has been shown to be a critical mediator of the host responses to a broad-spectrum of micro-organisms or microbial products (5-7,30,31,33). It also plays an important role in antigen-specific T cell activation and in the development of a humoral antibody response (34). MIF was reported to be an essential mediator of tuberculin-induced delayed-type hypersensitivity (52). A puzzling observation made during investigations of the biological activities of MIF was that physiological concentrations of glucocorticoids (dexamethasone or cortisol) induced MIF release from macrophages and T cells (33,34). Of note, glucocorticoid-induced macrophage MIF production followed a bell-shaped dose response curve with maximal release induced by concentrations of steroids in the range of 10^{-10}-10^{-14}M. However, at higher concentrations (10^{-6} M) dexamethasone was observed to inhibit MIF release. Moreover, the intravenous injection of dexamethasone increased the circulating concentrations of MIF in the rat (33). At first glance, these results appeared paradoxical and difficult to reconcile with the pro-inflammatory properties of MIF (5,6). Yet, this observation provided the impetus that led to the discovery that MIF functions as a counter-regulator of the anti-inflammatory effects of glucocorticoids. This intriguing property of MIF was revealed by the fact that adding recombinant MIF to human monocytes overcame in a dose-dependent fashion dexamethasone-induced inhibition of cytokine production (TNFα, IL-1β, IL-6 and IL-8) (33). MIF also was found to override dexamethasone-mediated suppression of T cell proliferation and cytokine production (IL-2 and IFNγ) stimulated by anti-CD3 antibodies (34).

Likewise, MIF overcame the anti-inflammatory effects of glucocorticoids on alveolar cells isolated from patients with ARDS (46).

In vivo, stress-induced activation of the HPA axis led to a rise of the serum MIF levels concomitant with the elevation of the blood concentrations of the stress-hormones ACTH and corticosterone (33). The counter-regulatory effect of MIF was confirmed in a mouse model of endotoxemia. Administration of MIF suppressed the protection conferred by glucocorticoids pre-treatment (33). Furthermore, median plasma concentrations of MIF are 3 ng/ml (i.e. 0.25 nM) (range: 1.9-5.4 ng/ml) at baseline (31), which is within the range of circulating levels of cortisol (10 nM). As noted for glucocorticoids, circulating concentrations of MIF also increase during inflammation, infection, or stress and thus may also exert modulatory activities during the acute phase of inflammatory or infectious diseases (31).

The observations that macrophage MIF production induced by microbial products and by glucocorticoids follows a bell-shaped curve and that its overriding capacity is reduced at high concentration of steroids imply the existence of numerous check points for MIF-glucocorticoid interactions. Taken together, these observations support the concept that MIF and glucocorticoids function as a physiological counter-regulatory dyad that controls host inflammatory and immune responses in the periphery and in the systemic circulation.

Glucocorticoids are known to inhibit cytokine production via an inhibition of gene transcription. The molecular mechanisms by which glucocorticoids exert these effects include the direct interaction between activated glucocorticoid receptors and the transcription NF-κB, AP-1 or CREB. Dexamethasone was reported to induce the transcription of the IkBα gene (53,54), thereby increasing IkBα protein concentrations in the cytoplasm and decreasing the amount of NF-κB translocating to the nucleus, leading to a reduction in cytokine production. Glucocorticoid-mediated effect on chromatin structure also may account for part of the anti-inflammatory effects of steroids. Glucocorticoids may bind to several transcription co-repressor molecules involved in histone deacetylase activity. The net effect is a tighter coiling of DNA that reduced the access of transcription factors to their specific binding sites, and thus result in the suppression of gene expression. Glucocorticoids may also reduce the stability of mRNA by binding to AU rich sequences in the 3' untranslated region of cytokine genes.

Little is known about the mechanisms underlying MIF overriding effects. However, two recent observations have shed some light on the mechanisms by which MIF may inhibit glucocorticoid-mediated effects. MIF was found to stimulate cytosolic phospholipase A_2 ($cPLA_2$) activity and arachidonic acid release by NIH-3T3 fibroblasts via a protein kinase A and p44/p42 extracellular signal-regulated (ERK) mitogen-activated protein kinase pathway (43). Given that $cPLA_2$ is the an important target of the anti-inflammatory action of glucocorticoids, the authors rightfully reasoned that $cPLA_2$ might be at the crossroad of opposing effects of MIF and glucocorticoids. In agreement with this hypothesis, recombinant MIF completely reversed the inhibitory effect of dexamethasone on arachidonic acid production by fibroblasts, providing a very plausible explanation as to how MIF may antagonize glucocorticoid action. Additional studies of the molecular basis of MIF-glucocorticoid interactions in the macrophage have revealed that MIF inhibits both transcriptional and post-transcriptional glucocorticoid-mediated suppression of pro-inflammatory gene expression (IL-8 and TNF) (T. Roger, manuscript in preparation).

The fact that MIF is located both centrally and in tissues in direct contact with the environment is consistent with its critical role in innate immune responses. In the periphery, the MIF produced by immune and epithelial cells in response to infectious stimuli would serve, in concert with other cytokines, to promote inflammatory and immune reactions to eliminate the invasive pathogen. By counteracting the anti-inflammatory and immunosuppressive effects of stress-induced augmentation of glucocorticoids, MIF specifically facilitates the development of primary host defenses. The release of pituitary MIF into the bloodstream also contributes to promote systemic innate and acquired immune responses.

CONCLUSIONS

Over the last decade, macrophage migration inhibitory factor (MIF) has emerged to be an important mediator of the innate immune system. Originally discovered as a T-cell cytokine, MIF was identified recently to be released by a vast array of cells, including immune (monocytes/macrophages, T cells, B cells, eosinophils, mast cells), endocrine (pituitary and adrenal cells) and epithelial cells in response to infection and stress. One important characteristic of MIF is the fact that it exists as a pre-formed intracellular protein, and is thus ready to be rapidly released when cells are activated. Bacteria, microbial toxins (LPS, TSST-1, SPEA) and cytokines (TNFα, IFNγ) were found to be powerful inducers of MIF secretion by monocytes and macrophages. High blood levels of MIF were measured in mice with bacterial peritonitis and in humans with severe sepsis and septic shock. Studies of experimental septic shock provided a direct evidence for an intrinsic contribution of MIF to the pathogenesis of sepsis. Immunoneutralization of MIF or deletion of the MIF gene protected mice against lethal endotoxemia, staphylococcal toxic shock and peritonitis induced by *E. coli* or cecal ligation and puncture. Noteworthy, anti-MIF antibodies were found to also protect TNFα knockout mice from lethal septic shock. Conversely, administration of recombinant MIF at the onset of endotoxemia or bacterial sepsis increased lethality, confirming the detrimental effects of excessive systemic levels of this pro-inflammatory mediator. MIF stimulates the expression of pro-inflammatory mediators by immune cells, and thus vigorously promotes inflammatory and immune responses. The surprising observations that MIF release was induced by glucocorticoids and that MIF had the unique feature to override the anti-inflammatory and immunosuppressive effects of glucocorticoids on macrophages and T-cells functions further emphasized the critical regulatory role played by MIF within the immune system. MIF and glucocorticoids appear to function as a physiological counter-regulatory dyad that modulates host inflammatory and immune responses. Given the central place of MIF in innate immune responses against infection and in the regulation of inflammatory responses, pharmacological modulation of MIF production or neutralization of MIF activity could have broad clinical applications and may offer new treatment options for the management of patients with severe sepsis, inflammatory and auto-immune diseases.

REFERENCES

1. Bloom BR, Bennett B. Mechanism of a reaction in vitro associated with delayed-type hypersensitivity. Science 1966;153:80-82.
2. David J. Delayed hypersensitivity in vitro: its mediation by cell-free substances formed by lymphoid cell-antigen interaction. PNAS 1966;56:72-77.
3. Calandra T, Bucala R. Macrophage migration inhibitory factor (MIF): a glucocorticoid counter-regulator within the immune system. Critical Reviews in Immunology 1997;17:77-88.
4. Weiser WY, Temple PA, Witek-Gianotti JS, Remold HG, Clark SC, David JR. Molecular cloning of a cDNA encoding a human macrophage migration inhibitory factor. PNAS 1989;86:7522-7526.
5. Bernhagen J, Calandra T, Mitchell RA, Martin SB, Tracey KJ, Voelter W, Manogue KR, Cerami A, Bucala R. MIF is a pituitary-derived cytokine that potentiates lethal endotoxaemia. Nature 1993;365:756-759.
6. Calandra T, Bernhagen J, Mitchell RA, Bucala R. The macrophage is an important and previously unrecognized source of macrophage migration inhibitory factor. J Exp Med 1994;179:1895-1902.
7. Bacher M, Meinhardt A, Lan HY, Metz CN, Chesney JA, Calandra T, Gemsa D, Donnelly T, Atkins RC, Bucala R. MIF expression in experimentally-induced endotoxemia. Am J Pathol 1997;150(1):235-246.

8. Bernhagen J, Calandra T, Bucala R. Regulation of the immune response by macrophage migration inhibitory factor: biological and structural features. J Mol Med 1998;76:151-161.
9. Swope MD, Lolis E. Macrophage migration inhibitory factor: cytokine, hormone, or enzyme? Rev Physiol Biochem Pharmacol 1999;139:1-32.
10. Paralkar V, Wistow G. Cloning the human gene for macrophage migration inhibitory factor (MIF). Genomics 1994;19: 48-51.
11. Mitchell R, Bacher M, Bernhagen J, Pushkarskaya T, Seldin M, Bucala R. Cloning and characterization of the gene for mouse macrophage migration inhibitory factor (MIF). J Immunol 1995;154:3863-3870.
12. Kozak CA, Adamson MC, Buckler CE, Segovia L, Paralkar V, Wistow G. Genomic cloning of mouse MIF (Macrophage Inhibitory Factor) and genetic mapping of the human and mouse expressed gene and nine mouse pseudogenes. Genomics 1995;27:405-411.
13. Bozza M, Kolakowski LF, Jenkins NA, Gilbert DJ, Copeland NG, David JR, Gerard C. Structural characterization and chromosomal location of the mouse macrophage migration inhibitory factor gene and pseudogenes. Genomics 1996;27:412-419.
14. Bozza M, Satoskar AR, Lin G, Lu B, Humbles AA, Gerard C, David JR. Targeted disruption of migration inhibitory factor gene reveals its critical role in sepsis. J Exp Med 1999;189(2):341-346.
15. Budarf M, McDonald T, Sellinger B, Kozak C, Graham C, Wistow G. Localization of the human gene for macrophage migration inhibitory factor (MIF) to chromosome 22q11.2. Genomics 1997;39(2):235-236.
16. Wistow GJ, Shaughnessy MP, Lee DC, Hodin J, Zelenka PS. A macrophage migration inhibitory factor is expressed in the differentiating cells of the eye lens. PNAS 1993;90:1272-1275.
17. Bernhagen J, Mitchell RA, Calandra T, Voelter W, Cerami A, Bucala R. Purification, bioactivity, and secondary structure analysis of mouse and human macrophage migration inhibitory factor (MIF). Biochemistry 1994;33:14144-14155.
18. Esumi N, Budarf M, Ciccarelli L, Sellinger B, Kozak CA, Wistow G. Conserved gene structure and genomic linkage for D-dopachrome tautomerase (DDT) and MIF. Mamm Genome 1998;9(9):753-757.
19. Waeber G, Thompson N, Chautard T, Steinmann M, Nicod P, Pralong FP, Calandra T, Gaillard RC. Transcriptional activation of the macrophage migration-inhibitory factor gene by the corticotropin-releasing factor is mediated by the cyclic adenosine 3',5'-monophosphate responsive element-binding protein CREB in pituitary cells. Mol Endocrinol 1998;12(5):698-705.
20. Ishizaka K, Ishii Y, Nakano T, Sugie K. Biochemical basis of antigen-specific suppressor T cell factors: controversies and possible answers. Adv Immunol 2000;74:1-60.
21. Sugimoto H, Taniguchi M, Nakagawa A, Tanaka I, Suzuki M, Nishihira J. Crystal structure of human D-dopachrome tautomerase, a homologue of macrophage migration inhibitory factor, at 1.54 A resolution. Biochemistry 1999;38(11):3268-3279.
22. Sun HW, Swope M, Cinquina C, Bedarkar S, Bernhagen J, Bucala R, Lolis E. The subunit structure of human macrophage migration inhibitory factor: evidence for a trimer. Protein Engineering 1996;9(8):631-635.

23. Suzuki M, Sugimoto H, Nakagawa A, Tanaka I, Nishihira J, Sakai M. Crystal structure of the macrophage migration inhibitory factor from rat liver. Nature Structural Biology 1996;3:259-266.
24. Subramanya HS, Roper DI, Dauter Z, Dodson EJ, Davies GJ, Wilson KS, Wigley DB. Enzymatic ketonization of 2-hydroxymuconate: specificity and mechanism investigated by the crystal structures of two isomerases. Biochemistry 1996;95(3):792-802.
25. Rosengren E, Bucala R, Åman P, Jacobsson L, Odh G, Metz CN, Rorsman H. The immunoregulatory mediator macrophage migration inhibitory factor (MIF) calalyzes a tautomerization reaction. Molecular Medicine 1996;2(1):143-149.
26. Rosengren E, Aman P, Thelin S, Hansson C, Ahlfors S, Björk P, Jacobsson L, Rorsman H. The macrophage migration inhibitory factor MIF is a phenylpyruvate tautomerase. FEBS Letters 1997;417:85-88.
27. Bendrat K, Al-Abed Y, Callaway DJE, Peng T, Calandra T, Metz CN, Bucala R. Biochemical and mutational investigations of the enzymatic activity of macrophage migration inhibitory factor. Biochemistry 1997;36(49):15356-15362.
28. Hermanowski-Vosatka A, Mundt SS, Ayala JM, Goyal S, Hanlon WA, Czerwinski RM, Wright SD, Whitman CP. Enzymatically inactive macrophage migration inhibitory factor inhibits monocyte chemotaxis and random migration. Biochemistry 1999;38(39):12841-12849.
29. Kleemann R, Kapurniotu A, Frank RW, Gessner A, Mischke R, Flieger O, Juttner S, Brunner H, Bernhagen J. Disulfide analysis reveals a role for macrophage migration inhibitory factor (MIF) as thiol-protein oxidoreductase. J Mol Biol 1998;280(1):85-102.
30. Calandra T, Spiegel LA, Metz CN, Bucala R. Macrophage migration inhibitory factor (MIF) is a critical mediator of the activation of immune cells by exotoxins of Gram-positive bacteria. PNAS 1998;95:11383-11388.
31. Calandra T, Echtenacher B, Roy DL, Pugin J, Metz CN, Hultner L, Heumann D, Mannel D, Bucala R, Glauser MP. Protection from septic shock by neutralization of macrophage migration inhibitory factor. Nat Med 2000;6(2):164-170.
32. Martiney JA, Sherry B, Metz CN, Espinoza M, Ferrer AS, Calandra T, Broxmeyer HE, Bucala R. Macrophage migration inhibitory factor release by macrophages after ingestion of plasmodium chabaudi-infected erythrocytes: possible role in the pathogenesis of malarial anemia. Infect Immun 2000;68(4):2259-2267.
33. Calandra T, Bernhagen J, Metz CN, Spiegel LA, Bacher M, Donnelly T, Cerami A, Bucala R. MIF as a glucocorticoid-induced modulator of cytokine production. Nature 1995;377:68-71.
34. Bacher M, Metz CN, Calandra T, Mayer K, Chesney J, Lohoff M, Gemsa D, Donnelly T, Bucala R. An essential regulatory role for macrophage migration inhibitory factor in T-cell activation. PNAS 1996;93:7849-7854.
35. Wymann D, Bluggel M, Kalbacher H, Blesken T, Akdis CA, Meyer HE, Blaser K. Human B cells secrete migration inhibition factor (MIF) and present a naturally processed MIF peptide on HLA-DRB1*0405 by a FXXL motif. Immunology 1999;96(1):1-9.
36. Takahashi A, Iwabuchi K, Suzuki M, Ogasawara K, Nishihira J, Onoé K. Antisense macrophage migration inhibitory factor (MIF) prevents anti-IgM mediated growth arrest and apoptosis of a murine B cell line by regulating cell cycle progression. Microbiol Immunol 1999;43(1):61-67.

37. Swope M, Sun H-W, Blake PR, Lolis E. Direct link between cytokine activity and a catalytic site for macrophage migration inhibitory factor. EMBO Journal 1998;17(13):3534-3541.
38. Makita H, Nishimura M, Miyamoto K, Nakano T, Tanino Y, Hirokawa J, Nishihira J, Kawakami Y. Effect of anti-macrophage migration inhibitory factor antibody on lipopolysaccharide-induced pulmonary neutrophil accumulation. Am J Respir Crit CareMed 1998;158:573-579.
39. Rossi AG, Haslett C, Hirani N, Greening AP, Rahman I, Metz CN, Bucala R, Donnelly SC. Human circulating eosinophils secrete macrophage migration inhibitory factor (MIF). Potential role in asthma. J Clin Invest 1999;101(12):2869-2874.
40. Chen H, Centola M, Altschul SF, Metzger H. Characterization of gene expression in resting and activated mast cells. J Exp:Med 1998;188(9):1657-1668.
41. Apte RS, Sinha D, Mayhew E, Wistow GJ, Niederkorn JY. Role of macrophage migration inhibitory factor in inhibiting NK cell activity and preserving immune privilege. J Immunol 1998;160(12):5693-5696.
42. Matsuda A, Tagawa Y, Matsuda H, Nishihira J. Identification and immunohistochemical localization of macrophage migration inhibitory factor in human cornea. FEBS Letters 1996;385:225-228.
43. Mitchell RA, Metz CN, Peng T, Bucala R. Sustained mitogen-activated protein kinase (MAPK) and cytoplasmic phopholipase A2 activation by macrophage migration inhibitory factor (MIF). J Biol Chem 1999;274(25):18100-18106.
44. Jüttner S, Bernhagen J, Metz CN, Röllinghoff M, Bucala R, Gessner A. Migration inhibitory factor induces killing of *Leishmania major* by macrophages: dependence on reactive nitrogen intermediates and endogenous TNF-α. J Immunol 1998;161:2383-2390.
45. Xu D, McSorley SJ, Tetley L, Chatfield S, Dougan G, Chan WL, Satoskar A, David JR, Liew FY. Protective effect on Leishmania major infection of migration inhibitory factor, TNF-alpha, and IFN-gamma administered orally via attenuated Salmonella typhimurium. J Immunol 1998;160(3):1285-1289.
46. Donnelly SC, Haslett C, Reid PT, Grant IS, Wallace WAH, Metz CN, Bruce LJ, Bucala R. Regulatory role for macrophage migration inhibitory factor in acute respiratory distress syndrome. Nat Med 1997;3(3):320-323.
47. Onodera S, Tanji H, Suzuki K, Kaneda K, Mizue Y, Sagawa A, Nishihira J. High expression of macrophage migration inhibitory factor in the synovial tissues of rheumatoid joints. Cytokine 1999;11(2):163-167.
48. Leech M, Metz C, Hall P, Hutchinson P, Gianis K, Smith M, Weedon H, Holdsworth SR, Bucala R, Morand EF. Macrophage migration inhibitory factor in rheumatoid arthritis: evidence of proinflammatory function and regulation by glucocorticoids. Arthritis Rheum 1999;42(8):1601-1608.
49. Metz CN, Bucala R. Role of macrophage migration inhibitory factor in the regulation of the immune response. Adv Immunol 1997;66:197-223.
50. Shimizu T, Abe R, Ohkawara A, Mizue Y, Nishihira J. Macrophage migration inhibitory factor is an essential immunoregulatory cytokine in atopic dermatitis. Biochem Biophys Res Commun 1997;240(1):173-178.
51. Nishino T, Bernhagen J, Shiiki H, Calandra T, Dohi K, Bucala R. Localization of macrophage migration inhibitory factor (MIF) to secretory granules within the corticotrophic and thyrotrophic cells of the pituitary gland. Mol Med 1995;1(7):781-788.

52. Bernhagen J, Bacher M, Calandra T, Metz CN, Doty SB, Donnelly T, Bucala R. An essential role for macrophage migration inhibitory factor in the tuberculin delayed-type hypersensitivity reaction. J Exp Med 1996;183:277-282.
53. Auphan N, DiDonato JA, Rosette C, Helmberg A, Karin M. Immunosuppression by glucocorticoids: inhibition of NF-kB activity trough induction of IkB synthesis. Science 1995;270:286-290.
54. Scheinman RI, Cogswell PC, Lofquist AK, Baldwin Jr AS. Role of transcriptional activation of IkBa mediation of immunosuppression by glucocorticoids. Science 1995;270:283-286.

Chapter 5

GENETIC SUSCEPTIBILITY TO INFECTION AND SEPSIS

Bradley D. Freeman, M.D.[†] and Barbara A. Zehnbauer, Ph.D.[‡]
Departments of Surgery[†] and Pathology[‡], Washington University School of Medicine, St. Louis, MO

Introduction

It is well accepted that an individual's genetic background plays an influential role in determining the susceptibility to, and outcome from, a variety of chronic illnesses. This is particularly true of many malignancies in which the precise relationships between genetic abnormalities and clinical manifestations have been abundantly described. In contrast, while intensivists have long appreciated that acutely ill individuals display enormous inter-patient variability in response to uniform insults, the possibility that genetic differences may be responsible for these individualized responses has largely been ignored. In this review, we will discuss recent studies that examine the clinical manifestations of acute illness in the context of genetic variants of the inflammatory and coagulation cascades. Ultimately, this gene-based approach will be essential to furthering our understanding of critical illness, identifying new therapeutic targets, and developing novel treatment strategies.

GENETIC PRINCIPLES USED IN THE ANALYSIS OF COMPLEX TRAITS

Clinical conditions such as sepsis pose several challenges to the investigator attempting to elucidate potential genetic mechanisms. Unlike diseases which are the result of a single genetic abnormality (e.g., cystic fibrosis or multiple endocrine neoplasia), the clinical presentation of more common "complex traits" is potentially influenced not only by multiple genes, but by innumerable environmental factors (e.g., the nature of infection, the specific antibiotics prescribed, the mode of mechanical ventilation employed, the patient's age and pre-morbid health, etc.) (1). Further, individuals affected by single-gene disorders with high penetrance, for example multiple endocrine neoplasia, will develop one or more clinical manifestations (>95%) and usually come to medical attention. This allows the medical geneticist to characterize the disorder, establish its mode of inheritance, and ultimately identify the abnormality at a molecular level. In contrast, individuals who are carriers for genetic variants related to increased risk of expression or predisposition to complex traits such as sepsis may be clinically unaffected until they encounter the appropriate environmental stimuli (e.g., trauma) or agent (drug). Further, unless several members of a family are exposed, the ability to infer a heritable component may be difficult to establish (2).

Attempts to understand the genetic background of complex traits have been aided immensely by recent characterization of DNA sequence polymorphisms. **Polymorphisms** are genetic variants present in the population at a frequency of greater than 1% (2). These polymorphisms exhibit Mendelian inheritance patterns, are widely distributed throughout the human genome, and have been instrumental in the construction of human genetic maps. Several types of polymorphic DNA markers have been described. **Restriction fragment length polymorphisms** (RFLP's) result from variations in DNA sequence that create or destroy specific cleavage sites for restriction endonucleases (2). This variability is detected as a change in the size of DNA fragments produced when DNA is reacted with restriction enzymes. This site alteration results in two different versions or alleles for the marker region (e.g., *Nco1* digestion producing TNF-α1 and TNF- α2 alleles, see below). Three different patterns are possible for a site polymorphism: two copies with the site (+/+), two copies lacking the site (-/-) (homozygotes), or a copy with and without the site (+/- or -/+) (e.g., heterozygote). Likewise, **variable number tandem repeats** (VNTR's), are length polymorphisms that differ by varying numbers of repeated copies of a consensus DNA sequence between two consistent restriction enzyme sites (2). As the number of repeated copies varies, a large number of differently sized polymorphic alleles result generating genetic heterozygosity. (See IL-1ra polymorphism below).

Traditionally, gene-disease correlations have been made by establishing the relationship between individuals manifesting the clinical condition (*phenotype*) and the polymorphic marker pattern (*genotype*) by pedigree analysis in family studies (2). Such linkage analysis reveals a physical proximity between the disease gene and the marker locus within a specific kindred (2). To determine the genetic contribution to a complex trait such as sepsis, familial inheritance patterns are not available (1). Thus, genetic linkage must be established by comparing gene frequencies in unrelated affected and unaffected individuals. Positive association in such studies is a concurrence between disease and marker alleles that is greater than predicted by chance (1). Because polymorphism frequencies are influenced by the ethnic composition of the study population, the composition of the healthy control population must be comparable to the diseased population.

THE ROLE OF GENETICS IN INFLUENCING THE OUTCOME TO INFECTION

The role of genetic background in determining the outcome to infection was suggested in an observational study examining the relative influences of inherited versus environmental factors in premature death (Table 1) (3). In this study, the causes of premature death of a large cohort of Danish adoptees were determined and broadly grouped into 3 categories: malignancy, vascular disease, and infection. To understand the relative influences of genetic versus environmental factors, these causes of death were compared with causes of premature death for both adoptive and biologic parents. Thus, premature death of biologic parents would be consistent with a strong genetic influence, while premature death of the adoptive parents would be consistent with a predominately environmental effect.

Table 1. Relative Influence of Biologic Versus Environmental Factors to Premature Death from Malignancy, Vascular Disease, and Infection in a Cohort of Adoptees

Cause of Death		Relative Risk	95% Confidence Interval
Malignancy	*Biologic*	1.19	0.16 - 8.99
	Adoptive	5.16	1.20 - 22.2
Vascular	*Biologic*	4.52	1.32 - 15.4
	Adoptive	3.02	0.72 - 12.8
Infectious	*Biologic*	5.81	2.47 - 13.7
	Adoptive	0.73	0.10 - 5.36

Modified from (3).

For adoptees whose biologic parents died prematurely of malignancy, the relative risk of premature cancer-related death was 1.19 (95% confidence interval: 0.16 to 8.99). In contrast, if the adoptive parents died prematurely of cancer, the relative risk of cancer-related death of the adoptees was 5.16

(95% confidence interval: 1.20 - 22.2). These findings suggest that the genetic contribution to cancer mortality was small overall, while the environmental contribution was substantial. In contrast, for adoptees whose biologic parents died prematurely of vascular disease, the relative risk of premature death was 4.52 (95% confidence interval: 1.32 - 15.4). In contrast, if the adoptive parents succumbed to vascular disease the relative risk was 3.02 (95% confidence interval: 0.72 - 12.8), suggesting in this study that genetics played a more prominent role than environmental factors. The most striking influence of genetic background, however, was observed for individuals dying prematurely of infection. If the adoptees' non-biologic parents succumbed prematurely to infectious causes, the relative risk of dying of infection was 0.73 (CI: 0.10 - 5.36). In contrast, if the adoptees biologic parents died prematurely of infection, the relative risk of premature death was 5.81 (CI: 2.47 - 13.7). Thus, among the causes of death considered, it appears that the strongest influence for genetic susceptibility to adverse outcome was from infectious causes. Since the publication of this article, the importance of genetics in determining the outcome for a variety of pathogens has been described, e.g., AIDS (4), hepatitis (5), and leishmaniasis (6). For the remainder of this chapter, we will focus on recent studies examining the importance of genetic background in influencing the outcome to sepsis and meningococcal infection.

TNF POLYMORPHISMS AND THE RISK OF INFECTION AND SEPSIS

A leading hypothesis of the pathogenesis of sepsis centers on the role of inflammation. According to this model, during severe infection, the primary host defense systems become overwhelmed, resulting in invasive infection and systemic release of pathogenic toxins. In response, host immune cells elaborate large quantities of both pro-and anti-inflammatory mediators. If left unchecked, this "excessive" inflammatory response is felt to result in shock, organ injury, and death (7). Tumor Necrosis Factor (TNF) is a prominent mediator of the sepsis response and a pivotal pro-inflammatory cytokine secreted in response to infectious challenge (7). Accordingly, genetic variants that modulate TNF expression or activity may potentially influence the clinical manifestations of sepsis for a given individual. The two principal forms of TNF, TNF-α and TNF-β bind the same receptors and may produce both similar and diverse biologic responses (8). In contrast to TNF-αwhich is expressed mainly by macrophages, TNF-β is expressed and released by lymphocytes (8). Genes encoding these cytokines are situated adjacently within the HLA class III genes on chromosome 6 (8). Recently, point mutations in both the TNF- αand TNF-β genes have been described which are associated with elevated levels of constitutive and inducible TNF secretion. For TNF-α, this site is located in the promoter region (position -308, e.g., 308 bp upstream from the transcriptional start of the genome) and results from a guanine (wild-type, TNF- α1) to adenine (TNF-α2) substitution (9). For TNF-β, this base change occurs in the first intron (position 1069), and results from an adenine (TNF-β 1) to guanine (TNF-β 2) change (9). While the mechanisms by which these genetic polymorphisms result in altered gene expression remain unclear, these variants have been implicated as having a pathogenic role in several infectious and inflammatory conditions (6). (Table 2).

Table 2: Summary of Polymorphisms of Common Mediators of the Inflammatory and Coagulation Pathways and their Disease Associations

Mediator	Polymorphism	Disease Associations	Clinical effect
TNF-α	Point mutation [G (TNF-α1) to (A(TNF-α2)] at position -308 TNF-α allele	Malaria (10)	TNF-α2 homozygotes at increased risk of cerebral malaria
	associated with increased TNF secretion	Meningococcus (11)	TNF-α2 allele associated with severe disease, death
		Sepsis (12)	TNF-α2 allele associated with increased mortality
TNF-β	Point mutation [A (TNF-β1) to (G (TNF-β2)] at position 1069	Sepsis (15)	TNF-β2 allele associated with increased mortality
	TNF-β2 allele associated with increased TNF secretion	Trauma (14)	TNF-β2 homozygotes at increased risk of severe sepsis
IL-1ra	Intron 2 contains variable number of 86 bp tandem repeats	Sepsis (15)	Frequency increased in septic patients
PAI-1	Insertion/deletion mutation (5G/4G) in promotor region. 4G mutation associated with elevated PAI-1 activity	Meningococcus (21,22)	4G/4G genotype associated with severe disease, mortality

Early studies attempting to understand the course of infectious illness in the context of TNF genotype focused on malaria and meningococcal disease (10,11). As with many infectious diseases, high circulating levels of TNF-α correlate with the severity of malarial infection, particularly cerebral involvement and adverse neurologic sequelae. It is hypothesized that TNF-α plays a pathogenic role in cerebral malaria, e.g., TNF-α induces upregulation of endothelial adhesion molecules that promote binding and vascular translocation of malarial parasites. Thus, individuals with genotypes associated with increased TNF-α secretion would be expected to experience more pronounced illness. In a large observational study undertaken in Gambia, it was found that individuals homozygous for the TNF-α2 genotype had a 4-fold increased risk of developing cerebral malaria, and a 7-fold increased risk of developing cerebral malaria with adverse neurologic sequelae, compared to individuals who were either heterozygous for this allele or who were of the wild-type genotype (10). A comparable finding was reported in children with meningococcal infection (11). Ninety-eight consecutive patients admitted to a pediatric intensive care unit in England with the diagnosis meningococcemia were genotyped. In this patient cohort, the TNF-α2 allele was associated with an increased risk of severe meningococcal disease (relative risk 1.6, odds ratio 1.1 to 2.3) and death (relative risk 2.5, odds ratio, 1.1 to 5.7) relative to the wild-type genotype (11). Of note, the frequency of the TNF-α2 allele in the healthy population in both of these studies was approximately 16% (10,11). Thus, while this allele appears pathologic in certain disease states, its maintenance in the gene pool suggests an important biologic role which, overall, compensates for these adverse effects.

Several recent population association studies have also examined the role of TNF genotype in influencing the outcome in patients with sepsis, septic shock, and trauma. Stuber *et al* genotyped 40 patients admitted to a German intensive care unit with the diagnosis of sepsis (12). Compared to individuals who were either wild-type or heterozygous for the TNF-α2 genotype, individuals homozygous for TNF-α2 developed much higher levels of circulating TNF-α ($p<0.004$) and had a much greater rate of mortality ($p=0.0022$). These results were confirmed in a larger multicenter French study by Mira *et al* (13). In this report, 89 patients with septic shock were genotyped and compared to non-septic patients in a case-control design. The TNF-α2 polymorphism frequencies differed significantly between these two groups (TNF-α2 frequency in septic patients was 39% vs. 18% in non-septic control patients, $p=0.002$) Further, mortality rates among carriers of the TNF-α2 allele was significantly higher than among patients with TNF-α

(71.4% vs. 42.6%, *p=0.008*). A similar finding was reported by Majetschak *et al* who examined the relationship between TNF-β genotype and the development of severe sepsis in a cohort of 110 patients following major blunt trauma (14). Individuals who were TNF-β 2 homozygotes were at significantly increased risk of developing severe sepsis, relative to individuals who were either carriers of this allele, or who had the wild-type genotype (Odds Ratio 3.07; 95% confidence interval 1.42 to 6.63). Corresponding to this finding, individuals who were TNF-β2 homozygotes had significantly higher levels of circulating TNF-α than did individuals with the other genotypes ($p<0.05$). Finally, Fang *et al* recently examined the relationship between TNF-β allele and outcome in a cohort of 93 patients with sepsis. The mortality for patients homozygous for the TNF-β2 allele was significantly higher (81%) than for either heterozygotes (42%) or wild-type individuals (19%) ($p<0.01$) (15). Collectively these studies suggest that TNF genotype influences both the susceptibility to, and severity of, sepsis and septic shock. These studies are summarized in Table 2.

GENETIC POLYMORPHISMS OF IL-1 AND IL-1RA AND OUTCOME IN SEPSIS

The Interleukin-1 (IL-1) family consists of 3 members: IL-1α, IL-1β, and IL-1 receptor antagonist (IL-1ra) (16). Both IL-1αand IL-1β function as pure agonists and produce a sepsis-like like picture when administered in animal models. In contrast, IL-1ra functions purely as an antagonist (16). Knock-out mice genetically deficient in IL-1ra have increased susceptibility to endotoxin induced lethality, while mice which over-express IL-1ra are relatively protected from endotoxin challenge (17). Thus, genetic variants which influence the circulating levels of either these agonistic or antagonistic inflammatory mediators may influence the outcome and severity of sepsis.

Intron 2 of the IL-1ra gene contains a variable number of 86bp tandem repeats. The corresponding alleles are termed A1, A2, A3, A4, A5 according the relative frequencies in healthy populations. Likewise, exon 5 of the IL-1β gene contains a polymorphic site for the restriction *Taq1*, defining two alleles (15). Fang *et al* examined the relationship between these IL-1β and IL-1ra polymorphisms and outcome from sepsis (15). Ninety three consecutive patients admitted to a German intensive care unit with sepsis were genotyped. Healthy blood donors served as controls. No differences were observed in the frequency of IL-1β polymorphisms comparing control and septic patients. In contrast, compared to controls, patients with sepsis had a significantly higher frequency of the IL-1raA2 allele. However, patients with the IL-1raA2 genotype did not differ in outcome relative to septic patients with other genotypes. Of note, there were 8 individuals in this study who were both carriers for IL-1raA2 and TNF-β2 homozygotes. All 8 of these individuals died of sepsis. While the size of this study was insufficient to draw conclusions about statistical associations, this particular genotype may identify an individual at particularly high risk for systemic inflammation and adverse outcome from sepsis. Consistent with this study, IL-1raA2 is associated with a number of chronic inflammatory disease including lichen sclerosis (18), lupus erythematosus (19), and ulcerative colitis (20). Thus, this allele may indicate increased susceptibility to inflammatory diseases, though the exact mechanism remains obscure.

GENETIC VARIATION IN THE FIBRINOLYSIS PATHWAY AND OUTCOME IN MENINGOCOCCAL DISEASE

Meningococcal infection continues to be a significantly morbid and potentially lethal disease. This pathogen characteristically elicits an intense inflammatory reaction which leads to endothelial injury, tissue damage, and organ dysfunction (21,22). Patients with fulminant meningococcal disease, e.g., septic shock or purpura fulminans, have evidence of activation of the coagulation cascade, with resulting disseminated intravascular coagulation, wide spread thrombosis, and tissue infarction (21,22). The pathophysiology of this procoagulant state is unclear and may result in part from an imbalance of pro- and anti-coagulant pathways as well as impairment of the fibrinolytic system (21,22).

Recently, interest has centered on the role of the serine protease plasminogen activator inhibitor-1 (PAI-1) in the pathogenesis of meningococcemia. PAI-1 is an acute phase reactant secreted by a variety of cell types in response to inflammatory stimuli (23). Preliminary studies suggest that circulating concentrations of PAI-1 are elevated in meningococcal infection, and correlate with disease severity and outcome (24). A common polymorphism has been identified in the promotor region of the PAI-1 gene resulting from a single base-pair insertion (5G)/deletion (4G)(25). The presence of guanine at position -675 in the 5G allele is essential for binding a repressor of transcriptase to the PAI-1 promotor (25). This may explain why *in vitro* models demonstrate that the presence of the 4G allele is associated with a 6-fold increase in PAI-1 expression in response to IL-1β relative to the wild-type allele. Similarly, individuals homozygous for the 4G allele have higher circulating basal and inducible concentrations of PAI-1 than individuals either heterozygous or homozygous than the 5G allele (25). Given the potential role for abnormalities of the fibrinolytic cascade to alter the course of meningococcal infection, studies have examined the impact of these polymorphisms on outcome from meningococcal disease.

To understand the potential influence of polymorphism of the PAI-1 gene in influencing the course of meningococcal disease, Hermans *et al*, genotyped a cohort of 123 pediatric patients admitted with the diagnosis of meningococcemia, and related this genotypic information to disease severity and course (21). Compared to control populations, the frequency of the various PAI-1 genotypes (e.g., 4G/4G, 4G/5G/ or 5G/5G) did not differ in patients with meningococcal disease, suggesting that PAI-1 was not important in determining susceptibility to this pathogen. Patients presenting with meningococcal disease had significantly higher concentrations of PAI-1 than control non-infected patients. Further, patients with more severe disease (e. g, sepsis or mixed sepsis/meningitis) had significantly higher PAI-1 concentrations than did patients with meningitis alone. Finally, patients with lethal meningococcal disease had higher concentrations of PAI-1 than did patients who survived, consistent with a potentially pathogenic role of PAI-1 in severe sepsis. Underlying these increases in PAI-1 levels was the finding that the 4G/4G genotype was associated with a significant increase in mortality rate relative to the other genotypes (relative risk of death 4.8, 95% confidence interval 1.8 to 13.0, $p=0.002$). These findings were confirmed in a second study by Westendorp *et al.* (22) who similarly demonstrated that patients with the 4G/4G genotype were significantly more likely to develop sepsis, than milder forms of meningococcal disease (odds ratio 5.9; 95% confidence interval: 1.9 to 18).

CONCLUSION

It is becoming increasingly apparent that an individual's genetic background may greatly influence the susceptibility to severe infection and/or the clinical course of sepsis. Much of the work in this area, to date, has focused on understanding the roles of functional genetic polymorphisms at a limited number of genetic loci (e.g., TNF-α, IL-1ra, PAI-1). While these studies have been informative, this approach is inherently limited. Specifically, the clinical manifestations of a disease such as sepsis will ultimately be dictated by multiple genes and numerous environmental factors. Further, while the presence or absence of specific polymorphisms may impact the course of acute illness, equally - if not more important - will be understanding the effects of combinations and sequences of gene expression in the acutely ill patient. Recent innovations in genomic technology, specifically the development of high volume rapid through-put assays (26,27), will dramatically expand the ability to understand critical illness at the genetic level. The ability to comprehensively genotype critically ill patients will allow investigators to understand the relationship between multiple genetic loci and physiologic response, how gene expression varies over the course of illness, and how complexes of genes are differentially expressed in functional compared with failing organs. Ultimately, such information will be essential to the identification of new therapeutic targets and the development of effective therapeutic strategies for the critically ill patient.

REFERENCES

1. Lander ES, Schork NJ. Genetic dissection of complex traits. Science. 1994;265:2037-48.
2. Zehnbauer BA, Romkes M, Carcillo JA. Textbook of Critical Care. In: Ayres SM, Grenvick A, Holbrook PR, Shoemaker WC, eds. Textbook of Critical Care. 4th ed. Philadelphia: W.B. Saunders Company; 1999.
3. Sorensen TIA, Nielsen GG, Anderson PK, Teasdale TW. Genetic and environmental influences on premature death in adult adoptees. N Engl J Med. 1988;318:727-32.
4. Winkler C, Modi W, Smith MW, et al. Genetic restriction of AIDS pathogenesis by an SDF-1 chemokine gene variant. Science. 1998;279:389-93.
5. Hohler T, Kruger A, Gerken G, Schneider PM, Buschenfelde KHMZ, Rittner C. A tumor necrosis factor-_ promotor polymorphism is associated with chronic hepatitis B infection. Clin Exp Immunol. 1998;111:579-82.
6. Cabrera M, Shaw MA, Sharples C, et al. Polymorphism in tumor necrosis factor genes associated with mucocutaneous Leishmaniasis. J Exp Med. 1995;182:1259-64.
7. Natanson C, Hoffman WD, Suffredini AF, Eichacker PQ, Danner RL. Selected treatment strategies for septic shock based on proposed mechanisms of pathogenesis. Ann Int Med. 1994;120:771-83.
8. Nedwin GE, Naylor SL, Sakaguchi AY. Human lymphotoxin and tumor necrosis factor genes: structure, homology, and chromosomal localization. Nuc Acid Res. 1985;13:6351-73.
9. Pociot F, Briant L, Jongeneel CV. Association of tumor necrosis factor (TNF) and class II major histocompatibility complex alleles with the secretion of TNF-alpha and TNF-beta by human mononuclear cells: a possible link to insulin-dependent diabetes mellitus. Eur J Immunol. 1993;23:224-31.
10. McGuire W, Hill AVS, Allsopp CEM, Greenwood BM, Kwiatkowski D. Variation in the TNF promotor region associated with susceptibility to cerebral malaria. Nature. 1994;371:508-11.
11. Nadel S, Newport MJ, Booy R, Levin M. Variation in the tumor necrosis factor gene promotor region may be associated with death from meningococcal disease. J Infect Dis. 2000;174:878-80.
12. Stuber F, Peterson M, Bokelmann F, Schade U. A genomic polymorphism with in the tumor necrosis factor locus influences plasma tumor necrosis factor concentrations and outcome of patients with severe sepsis. Crit Care Med. 1996;24:381-4.
13. Mira, J. P., Cariou, A., Grall, F., Delclaux, C., Losser, M. R., Heshmati, F., Cheval, C., Monchi, M., Teboul, J. L., Riche, F., Leleu, G., Arbibe, L., Mignon, A., Delpech, M., and Dhainaut, J. P. Association of TNF2, a TNF promotor polymorphism, with septic shock susceptibility and mortality - a multicenter study. JAMA 282(6), 561-568. 8-11-1999.

14. Majetschak M, Flohe S, Obertacke U, et al. Relation of a TNF gene polymorphism to severe sepsis in trauma patients. Ann Surg. 1999;230:207-14.
15. Fang XM, Schroder S, Hoeft A, Stuber F. Comparison of two polymorphisms of the interleukin-1 gene family: interleukin-1 receptor antagonist polymorphism contributes to susceptibility to severe sepsis. Crit Care Med. 1999;27:1330-4.
16. Dinarello CA. Is there an interleukin-1 genetic predisposition to developing severe sepsis? Crit Care Med. 1999;27:1397-8.
17. Hirsch E, Irikura VM, Paul SM. Functions of interleukin-1 receptor antagonist in gene knock-out and over-producing mice. PNAS 1996;93:11008-13.
18. Clay FE, Cork MJ, Tarlow JK. Interleukin-1 receptor antagonist gene polymorphism association with lichen sclerosis. Hum Genet. 1994;94:407-10.
19. Blakemore AI, Tarlow JK, Cork MJ. Interleukin-1 receptor antagonist gene polymorphism as a disease severity factor in systemic lupus erythematosus. Arthrit Rheum. 1994;37:1380-5.
20. Mansfield JC, Holden H, Tarlow JK. Novel genetic association between ulcerative colitis and the anti-inflammatory cytokine interleukin-1 receptor antagonist. Crit Care Med. 1994;106:637-42.
21. Hermans PWM, Hibberd ML, Booy R, et al. 4G/5G promotor polymorphism in the plasminogen-activator inhibitor-1 gene and outcome of meningococcal disease. Lancet. 1999;354:556-600.
22. Westendorp RGJ, Hottenga JJ, Slagboom PE. Variation in plasminogen-activator-inhibitor-1 gene and risk of meningococcal septic shock. Lancet. 1999;354:561-3.
23. Pannekoek H, Veerman H, Lambers H. Endothelial plasminogen activator-1: a new member of the serpin gene family. EMBO J. 1986;5:2539-44.
24. Kornelisse RF, Hazelzet JA, Savelkoul HFJ. The relationship between plasminogen activator-1 and pro-inflammatory and counter-inflammatory mediators in children with meningococcal septic shock. J Infect Dis. 1996;173:1148-56.
25. Dawson SJ, Wiman B, Hamsten A, Green F, Humphries S, Henney AM. The two allele sequences of a common polymorphism in the promotor of the plasminogen activoator-1 (PAI-1) gene respond differently to interleukin-1 in HEPG2 cells. J Biol Chem. 1993;268:10739-45.
26. Service RF. Microchip arrays put DNA on the spot. Science. 1998;282:396-9.
27. Chen X, Zehnbauer B, Gnirke A, Kwok P-Y. Fluorescence energy transfer detection as a homogeneous DNA diagnostic method. PNAS. 1997;94:10756-61.

Chapter 6

IMPACT OF GENOMIC VARIATIONS ON INFLAMMATORY PROCESSES AND SEPSIS

Frank Stüber, M.D.
University of Bonn, Department of Anesthesiology and Critical Care Medicine, Bonn, Germany

Introduction

The immune response to injury involves a complex pattern of primary, secondary and tertiary humoral and cellular responses. Genetic variability in the expression of the mediators comprising these responses constitutes the genetic background which may potentially influence the course of inflammation in each individual. Differences in this background may in part explain the highly variable clinical courses noted among septic patients. Comparable doses of infecting microbes may induce a wide range of severity of illness due in part to genetic variability.

Endotoxin, a constituent of cell walls of gram-negative bacteria, appears to be a major inducer of inflammatory responses in human infections. Both exogenous microbial organisms infecting the human organism as well as the large endogenous pool of bacteria within the human gastrointestinal tract may contribute to the release of endotoxin and other toxins which challenge the human immune system in differing states of disease (2).

Primary responses in inflammation are mediated by proinflammatory cytokines such as tumor necrosis factor (TNF) and interleukin 1 (IL-1) (3). Secondary proinflammatory mediators like interleukin 6 (IL-6) and interleukin 8 (IL-8) as well as antiinflammatory cytokines like interleukin-1 receptor antagonist (IL-1ra) and interleukin-10 (IL-10) are induced by TNF and IL-1 (3). Tertiary mediators comprise factors of different, even non-cytokine origin such as proteases, coagulation factors, kinins, eicosanoids, nitric oxide and others which effects the distal part of mediator cascades (4).

Recent evidence suggests that proinflammatory mediators like TNF may also stimulate the production of antiinflammatory mediators with important effects on the host's immune system (5). Antiinflammatory mediators induce a state of immunosuppression in sepsis which has also been named immunoparalysis (6). This state of decreased immunoreactivity is accompanied by high levels of antiinflammatory cytokines such as IL-10 and interleukin –1 receptor antagonist (IL-1ra) (7). It also includes a decrease in the number of expressed surface HLA class II molecules on circulating monocytes/macrophages and impaired ex vivo responses of peripheral blood leukocytes to lipopolysaccharide (LPS) (8).

Thus, both pro- and antiinflammatory responses contribute to the overall outcome of patients with systemic inflammation and sepsis. Therefore, all genes encoding proteins involved in the transduction of inflammatory processes are candidate genes determining the human genetic background responsible for interindividual differences in systemic inflammatory responses to injury. Genetically determined differences in cytokine production and release, heat shock protein expression, nitric oxide synthase activity or coagulation factor as well as other inflammatory mediators may contribute to the wide range of clinical manifestations observed in patients with inflammatory disease: For example, a patient with peritonitis may present without symptoms of sepsis and recover within days or may suffer from fulminant septic shock resulting in death within hours.

Recognizing the genetic background constituting each individual's inflammatory response to infectious as well as noninfectious challenges is important for several reasons. First, it will provide information for basic science concerning the role and interaction of mediators. Second, and more important, clinically it will help identify patients at greatest risk of developing severe sepsis and multiple organ dysfunction during a systemic inflammatory reaction. This will in turn help determine those least likely to survive. Based on this information it may be possible to predict which patients will benefit most from anti-mediator strategies.

CANDIDATE GENES

One goal in determining the role of the genetic background in inflammatory responses is to identify genomic markers suitable for clinical use and risk stratification of patients. Another goal is to understand the influence of genomic variations on gene regulation and protein expression. Because members of the cytokine family like tumor necrosis factor are highly conserved in evolution (9), cytokine research has concentrated on the study of the structure and function of single genes which clearly contribute to disease. Few genomic polymorphisms for cytokines are presently recognized and the functional relevance of identified genomic variations remains unclear.

PROINFLAMMATORY CYTOKINES

Primary proinflammatory cytokines like TNF and IL-1 induce secondary pro- and antiinflammatory mediators like IL-6 and IL-10. They have been shown to contribute substantially to the host's primary response to infection. Both, TNF and IL-1, are capable of inducing the same symptoms and the same severity of septic shock and organ dysfunction as endotoxin in experimental settings as well as in humans (10). Genetic variations in the TNF and IL-1 genes are of major interest given the influences they might have in determining the host's response to endotoxin.

Tumor Necrosis Factor

TNF is considered to be one of the most important mediators of endotoxin induced effects. Interindividual differences in TNF release have been described (11,12). The TNF locus consists of three functional genes. TNF is positioned between lymphotoxin α (LTα) in the upstream direction and lymphotoxin β (LTβ) in the downstream direction. Genomic polymorphisms within in the TNF locus have been under intense investigation. Genetic variation within the TNF locus is rare as the TNF gene is well conserved throughout evolution (9). The coding region of this gene is especially highly conserved.

Much interest has been focused on the genomic variations of the TNF locus. Biallelic polymorphisms defined by restriction enzymes (NcoI, AspHI) or other single base changes (-308, -238) as well as multiallelic microsatellites (TNFa-e) have been investigated in *in vitro* studies and in various diseases in which TNF is considered to have an important pathogenic role. The functional importance of TNF gene regulation has been suggested by two polymorphisms within the TNF promoter region. Single base changes have been detected at –850, –376, -308 and position -238 (13-16). A G to A transition at position -308 has been associated with susceptibility to cerebral malaria (17). These results could not be confirmed however by another malaria study which showed fewer febrile episodes in heterozygous carriers of the allele TNF2 (18) The rare allele TNF2 (A at position -308) was suggested to be linked to high TNF promoter activity (17). Autoimmune diseases like diabetes mellitus or lupus erythematosus did not show differences in allele frequencies or genotype distribution between patients and controls (19,20). In addition, patients with severe sepsis and a high proportion of gram-negative infections also did not display altered allele frequencies associated with either promoter polymorphisms (position -238 and -308) (21). Analysis of the TNF promoter by means of reporter gene constructs revealed contradictory results: A first report showed a functional role of a –308 G to A transition (17). Two papers could not confirm differences of the TNF promoter activity in relation to the -308 polymorphism (21,22). A recent paper reports on a possible influence of TNF promoter activity by the -308 G to A transition in a B cell line (23). Genotyping of this polymorphism in patients with severe sepsis did not contribute to risk assessment. The -308 polymorphism did not appear to be a marker for susceptibility to nor outcome of severe sepsis caused by gram-negative infection (21). Also, TNF plasma levels do not seem to be influenced by this polymorphism in patients with severe abdominal sepsis (Fig.1).

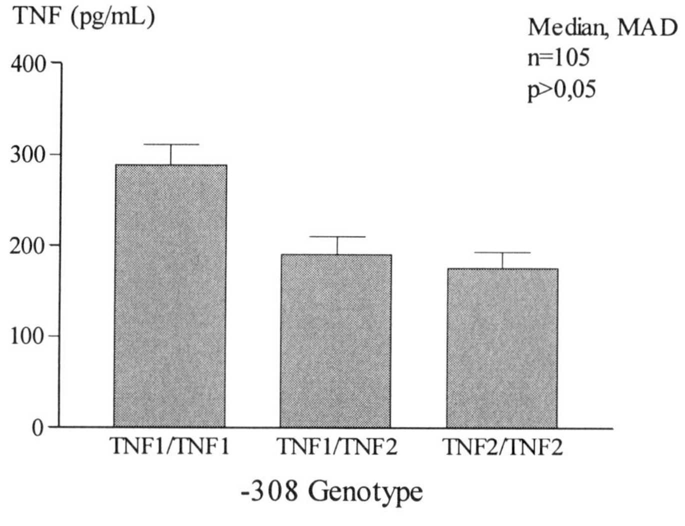

Figure 1. Median (median absolute deviation, MAD) of TNF plasma levels in 105 patients with severe sepsis grouped according to their –308 TNF promoter genotype (TNF1: Guanine; TNF2: Adenine)

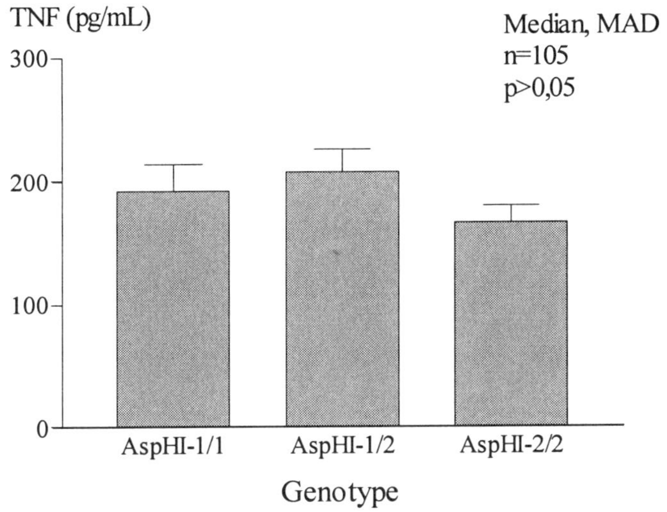

Figure 2: Median (median absolute deviation, MAD) of TNF plasma levels in 105 patients with severe sepsis grouped according to their AspHI genotype (Intron 1 of Lymphotoxin-α)

Despite the above findings, the results of a recent study did suggest an association of the rare allele TNF2 with non-survivors of septic shock (24). This publication again opens the discussion about the functionality of the –308 TNF promoter polymorphism and its possible relevance for routine clinical use. Differences in the results from these studies emphasize the need for formal standards of genotyping techniques have to be established. Do some typing techniques like allele-specific amplification result in over- or underestimation of certain alleles and genotypes?

Compared to genomic variations located in the promoter region, the functional relevance of intronic polymorphisms appear even less clear. Two biallelic polymorphisms located within intron two of LTα have been studied in autoimmune disease (25,26). One polymorphism is characterized by absence or presence of an NcoI restriction site. First reports demonstrated genomic blots revealing characteristic 5.5 or 10.5 kb bands after genomic NcoI digestion which hybridize to TNF specific probes (27). These bands correspond to the presence and absence, respectively, of an NcoI restriction site within intron one of lymphotoxin-α (LTα).

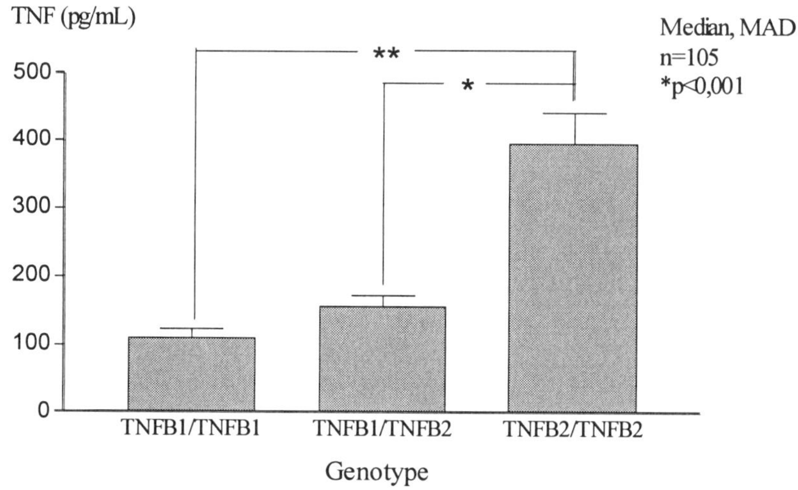

Figure 3. Median (median absolute deviation, MAD) of TNF plasma levels in 105 patients with severe sepsis grouped according to their Lymphotoxin-α (TNFβ) NcoI genotype.

The allele TNFB2 of this NcoI polymorphism (10.5 kb band) has been shown to be associated with high TNFα release ex vivo (28). Other studies showed no differences between genotypes in other models of ex vivo TNF induction while another study suggests an increased LTα response in TNFB2 homozygotes (12). Determination of which genotype is associated with a high proinflammatory response during severe gram-negative infection and severe sepsis can not yet be answered by *ex vivo* studies, however. Variability in cell culture and cytokine induction methods may contribute to differing results. In addition, the genomic NcoI polymorphism within intron one of the LTα gene may represent a genomic marker not directly related to overall gene regulation. However, this genomic marker may be associated with as yet undetected genomic variations which are responsible for genetic determination of high proinflammatory responses. Results from studies in patients with severe intraabdominal sepsis suggest TNFB2 homozygotes are associated with a high TNF response (Fig. 3). In contrast, genotyping for another biallelic polymorphism within intron 1 of LTα (AspHI) did not show significant association with TNF plasma levels (Fig. 2).

Several studies in chronic inflammatory autoimmune diseases suggest an association between TNFB2 and the incidence or severity and outcome of the disease (25,26,29). Studies in acute inflammatory diseases like severe sepsis in patients on surgical intensive care units showed a correlation between TNFB2 homozygosity and mortality (21) and the incidence of septic states in traumatized patients (30). TNFB2 homozygotes displayed a relative risk of 2.9 of dying from severe sepsis when compared to corresponding genotypes.

Interleukin-1

Besides TNF, IL-1 is another potent proinflammatory cytokine released by macrophages in the systemic inflammatory response. IL-1 is capable of inducing the symptoms of septic shock and organ failure in animal models and is regarded as a primary mediator of the systemic inflammatory response. Antagonizing IL-1 in endotoxin challenged animals including primates abrogates the lethal effects of endotoxin (31). A biallelic TaqI polymorphism has been described within the coding region (exon 5) of IL-1β (32,33). Despite the finding that a homozygous TaqI genotype correlates with high IL-1β secretion (32), genotyping of patients with severe sepsis did not reveal any association with incidence or outcome of disease.

Interleukin-6

IL-6 is a secondary cytokine with important immunologic functions like enhancement of B lymphocyte proliferation. It is released by macrophages and endothelial cells. Although direct toxic effects mediated by IL-6 in severe sepsis and septic shock have not been demonstrated yet, the proinflammatory activity is obvious. IL-6 has gained importance as a new clinical parameter for monitoring inflammatory activity in the course of acute inflammatory diseases. Studies testing the anti-TNF monoclonal antibody approach in the treatment of severe sepsis have used IL-6 levels as a marker of severe inflammation to randomize patients (34).

Genomic polymorphisms of the IL-6 gene have been described in the 3′ flanking region (35). In addition, two single base changes have been reported for the MspI and BcgII restriction site (36, 37).

Studies have thus far not shown an association between genomic variation of IL-6 and autoimmune diseases like lupus erythematosus (38). Functional studies concerning the influence of genomic variations on gene transcription or mRNA stability do not exist. In another study, allele frequencies and genotype distributions of the BcgII biallelic polymorphism did not differ in patients with rheumatoid arthritis compared to normal controls (29). Despite the apparent association between IL-6 levels and outcome in sepsis, studies assessing the possible difference in genomic variation on IL-6 in sepsis have not yet been done.

ANTIINFLAMMATORY CYTOKINES

Interleukin-1 Receptor Antagonist

Proinflammatory mediators comprise the hyperinflammatory side of the systemic inflammatory reaction. At the same time, antiinflammatory mediators are induced by proinflammatory cytokines and act to counterbalance the inflammatory response. Release of antiinflammatory mediators may also be excessive, however. Antiinflammatory proteins like IL-4, IL-10, IL-11 or IL-13 or IL-1ra may contribute to a very powerful downregulation of cellular and humoral proinflammatory activities. This downregulation results in decreased expression of class II molecules in antigen presenting cells as well as in low ex vivo responses of immuncompetent cells to inflammatory stimuli. This state of immunosuppression has also been termed immunoparalysis and may compromise host defense (6). This has been termed a compensatory antiinflammatory response syndrome (CARS) (39). Thus, genetic predisposition to an overproduction of these antiinflammatory mediators may be just as detrimental to outcome as one causing excessive proinflammatory mediator release.

A genomic polymorphism of the antiinflammatory cytokine IL-1ra has been identified within intron two and consists of variable numbers of a tandem repeat (VNTR) of a 86 bp motif. This 86 basepair motif contains at least three known binding sites for DNA binding proteins (40). Ex vivo experiments suggest higher IL-1ra responses combined with alleles containing low numbers of the 86 bp repeat. Ex vivo studies also demonstrate a higher level of IL-1ra protein expression and protein release in A2 homozygous individuals compared to heterozygotes following stimulation with lipopolysaccharide (41).

The allele A2 has been associated with the incidence of autoimmune diseases like lupus erythematosus and insulin dependent diabetes mellitus (42, 43). To date, however, no such differences appear to exist for surviving or non-surviving patients with severe sepsis. This finding is in contrast to the results concerning the biallelic NcoI polymorphism within intron one of LTα: Homozygotes for the TNFB2 genotype revealed a high mortality when compared to heterozygotes and TNFB1 homozygotes. The overall group of patients with severe sepsis did not show an increase in the TNFB2 allele frequency. For the IL-1ra polymorphism, however, an increase of the allele A2 in the patients with severe sepsis was detected. Patients carrying the haplotype TNFB2 homozygous and A2 homozygous did not survive in this study.

OTHER CANDIDATE GENES

Besides cytokines, several noncytokine host molecules are known to contribute to the toxicity associated with endotoxin. These include nitric oxide (NO), eicosanoids, platelet activating factor (PAF), coagulation cascade products, and heat shock proteins (44-46).

Nitric Oxide and NO-Synthase

Excessive release of nitric oxide has been closely associated with the hypotension occurring in severe sepsis and septic shock. Endotoxin and proinflammatory mediators like TNF and IL-1 stimulate an inducible form of NO-synthase (iNOS2) in macrophages and the vascular endothelium (47). In macrophages, NO is a potent radical and contributes to killing of invading pathogens. Pharmacological antagonism of NO synthesis reverses hypotension in animal models of septic shock as well as in patients (48).

Constitutive and inducible isoforms of NOS exist and are regulated differently. Some constitutively expressed forms are tissue specific (brain, neuron, vessels) while inducible forms are expressed in endothelial cells and macrophages. A single base change has been discovered in the promoter region of the human endothelial NO-synthase (NOS3). This polymorphism has been associated with the risk of coronary artery disease related to smoking (49). However, there is a lack of studies examining NOS3 promoter activities and NOS3 expression depending on allele and genoype. Associations between NOS polymorphisms and the incidence or outcome of septic shock have not been reported yet.

Heat shock Protein Genes

Heat shock proteins represent a physiologic response to cellular stress which is highly conserved in evolution. Heat shock proteins act as molecular chaperones and facilitate this intracellular folding of synthesized proteins (46). Inhibition of the heat shock response worsens septic shock in animal models. Induction of heat shock proteins prior to lethal endotoxin challenges reduces the lethality of septic shock (46).

A well studied member of the heat shock protein family is HSP 70. Two genomic polymorphisms have been described within the HSP 70-2 and the HSP 70 HOM gene. The first is an inducible form of HSP while the latter is expressed constitutively (50). No study testing the relation between allele and HSP 70-HOM expression has been performed. The HSP 70-2 polymorphism has been related to variable expression of HSP 70-2 mRNA

(51). Thus, the functional relevance of these HSP polymorphisms still has to be elucidated.

Genotyping of heat shock proteins in patients with severe sepsis does not show significant differences in allele frequencies or genotype distribution compared to healthy controls. On the other hand, a significant linkage between HSP 70-2/2 homozygotes and TNFB2 homozygotes was demonstrated (data not shown). In this context, the allele HSP 70-2/2 may be included in an extended haplotype of several alleles linked to each other and defining individuals at risk for developing or even dying from severe sepsis.

From Flies to Mice to Man

Mechanisms for the transduction of the LPS signal into the cell have recently been identified. An analogon of the so called toll receptor in the drosophila species which transduces signals for the elaboration of innate immune responses directed against bacteria and fungi has been identified in mice and other species (52). A single base pair change resulting in an amino acid alteration of the murine toll like receptor 4 (TLR4) renders the extensively studied mouse strain CH3/HeJ highly resistant to LPS challenge (53). Nine toll-like receptors (TLR1-9) (54) have been identified in mammals so far. TLR1, 3 and 5-9 have been found to be orphan receptors, whereas TLR2 has been shown to transduce peptidoglykan stimulation by gram-positive organisms (55-57). In contrast, TLR4 seems to play a key role in the LPS-induced signaling pathway (58-61).

From the historical perspective, the first evidence for a genetic predisposition to sepsis emerged from an experiment of nature, the discovery of the endotoxin-resistant mouse. The genetic locus of this endotoxin resistance (denoted *lps*) has been mapped to mouse chromosome 4 (58) and a functionally significant gene and product have been identified (TLR4). Presence of a functional TLR4 gene and gene product appears to be one of several determinants of outcome in endotoxemia. Survey of inbred laboratory mice demonstrated a broad range of sensitivity to endotoxin, and genetic analysis of inbred recombinant mice (genetically defined crosses of the most and least sensitive of the laboratory strains) demonstrates five loci that appeared to regulate endotoxin sensitivity. High resolution mapping is in progress. The data suggests that response to endotoxemia is a definable multigenic characteristic of laboratory mice. In humans, the work of Beutler and colleagues reveals several genomic variations within the coding region of human TLR4 (53). It still remains to be evaluated, whether the function of the human TLR4 is affected by these polymorphisms. However, if this is the case, the gene for the human TLR4 may be a very important candidate gene for studies to determine the genomic contribution to variability of innate immunity.

Conclusions

Understanding the influence genetic predisposition has on the inflammatory process may provide a basis for developing valuable diagnostic tools and new therapeutic approaches in severe sepsis. Evaluation of possible genomic markers for risk stratification of septic patients has just begun. Many candidate genes still have to be studied and the clinical significance of genomic markers must still be tested. This new approach may ultimately provide entry criteria for studies testing immunomodulatory agents in severe sepsis.

REFERENCES:

1. Sasse KC, Nauenberg E, Long A, Anton B, Tucker HJ, Hu TW. Long-term survival after intensive care unit admission with sepsis. Crit Care Med 1995;23:1040-1047.
2. Edmiston CE, Jr., Condon RE. Bacterial translocation. Surg Gynecol Obstet 1991;173:73-83.
3. Blackwell TS, Christman JW. Sepsis and cytokines. current status. Br J Anaesth 1996;77:110-117.
4. Bernard GR, Wheeler AP, Russell JA, Schein R, Summer WR, Steinberg KP, Fulkerson WJ, Wright PE, Christman BW, Dupont WD, Higgins SB, Swindell BB. The effects of ibuprofen on the physiology and survival of patients with sepsis. The Ibuprofen in Sepsis Study Group. N Engl J Med 1997;336:912-918.
5. van der Poll T, de Waal Malefyt R, Coyle SM, Lowry SF. Antiinflammatory cytokine responses during clinical sepsis and experimental endotoxemia: sequential measurements of plasma soluble interleukin (IL)-1 receptor type II, IL-10, and IL-13. J Infect Dis 1997;175:118-122.
6. Volk HD, Reinke P, Krausch D, Zuckermann H, Asadullah K, Muller JM, Docke WD, Kox WJ. Monocyte deactivation--rationale for a new therapeutic strategy in sepsis. Intensive Care Med 1996;22 Suppl 4:S474-81:S474-81.
7. Fisher CJ, Jr., Slotman GJ, Opal SM, Pribble JP, Bone RC, Emmanuel G, Ng D, Bloedow DC, Catalano MA. Initial evaluation of human recombinant interleukin-1 receptor antagonist in the treatment of sepsis syndrome: a randomized, open- label, placebo-controlled multicenter trial. The IL-1RA Sepsis Syndrome Study Group. Crit Care Med 1994;22:12-21.
8. Docke WD, Randow F, Syrbe U, Krausch D, Asadullah K, Reinke P, Volk HD, Kox W. Monocyte deactivation in septic patients: restoration by IFN- gamma treatment. Nat Med 1997;3:678-681.
9. Gray PW, Aggarwal BB, Benton CV, Bringman TS, Henzel WJ, Jarrett JA, Leung DW, Moffat B, Ng P, Svedersky LP, et al. Cloning and expression of cDNA for

human lymphotoxin, a lymphokine with tumour necrosis activity. Nature 1984;312:721-724.

10. Weinberg JR, Boyle P, Meager A, Guz A. Lipopolysaccharide, tumor necrosis factor, and interleukin-1 interact to cause hypotension. J Lab Clin Med 1992;120:205-211.
11. Westendorp RG, Langermans JA, Huizinga TW, Elouali AH, Verweij CL, Boomsma DI, Vandenbrouke JP. Genetic influence on cytokine production and fatal meningococcal disease. Lancet 1997;349:170-173.
12. Whichelow CE, Hitman GA, Raafat I, Bottazzo GF, Sachs JA. The effect of TNF*B gene polymorphism on TNF-alpha and -beta secretion levels in patients with insulin-dependent diabetes mellitus and healthy controls. Eur J Immunogenet 1996;23:425-435.
13. Kato T, Honda M, Kuwata S, Juji T, Kunugi H, Nanko S, Fukuda M, Honda Y. Novel polymorphism in the promoter region of the tumor necrosis factor alpha gene: No association with narcolepsy. Am J Med Genet 1999;88:301-304.
14. Knight JC, Udalova I, Hill AV, Greenwood BM, Peshu N, Marsh K, Kwiatkowski D. A polymorphism that affects OCT-1 binding to the TNF promoter region is associated with severe malaria. Nat Genet 1999;22:145-150.
15. Wilson AG, di Giovine FS, Blakemore AI, Duff GW. Single base polymorphism in the human tumour necrosis factor alpha (TNF alpha) gene detectable by NcoI restriction of PCR product. Hum Mol Genet 1992;1:353-353.
16. Brinkman BM, Huizinga TW, Kurban SS, van der Velde EA, Schreuder GM, Hazes JM, Breedveld FC, Verweij CL. Tumour necrosis factor alpha gene polymorphisms in rheumatoid arthritis: association with susceptibility to, or severity of, disease? Br J Rheumatol 1997;36:516-521.
17. McGuire W, Hill AV, Allsopp CE, Greenwood BM, Kwiatkowski D. Variation in the TNF-alpha promoter region associated with susceptibility to cerebral malaria. Nature 1994;371:508-510.
18. Stirnadel HA, Stockle M, Felger I, Smith T, Tanner M, Beck HP. Malaria infection and morbidity in infants in relation to genetic polymorphisms in Tanzania. Trop Med Int Health 1999;4:187-193.
19. Pociot F, Wilson AG, Nerup J, Duff GW. No independent association between a tumor necrosis factor-alpha promotor region polymorphism and insulin-dependent diabetes mellitus. Eur J Immunol 1993;23:3050-3053.
20. Wilson AG, Gordon C, di Giovine FS, de Vries N, van de Putte LB, Emery P, Duff GW. A genetic association between systemic lupus erythematosus and tumor necrosis factor alpha. Eur J Immunol 1994;24:191-195.
21. Stuber F, Udalova IA, Book M, Drutskaya LN, Kuprash DV, Turetskaya RL, Schade FU, Nedospasov SA. -308 tumor necrosis factor (TNF) polymorphism is not associated with survival in severe sepsis and is unrelated to lipopolysaccharide inducibility of the human TNF promoter. J Inflamm 1995;46:42-50.
22. Brinkman BM, Zuijdeest D, Kaijzel EL, Breedveld FC, Verweij CL. Relevance of the tumor necrosis factor alpha (TNF alpha) -308 promoter polymorphism in TNF alpha gene regulation. J Inflamm 1995;46:32-41.
23. Wilson AG, Symons JA, McDowell TL, McDevitt HO, Duff GW. Effects of a polymorphism in the human tumor necrosis factor alpha promoter on transcriptional activation. Proc Natl Acad Sci USA 1997;94:3195-3199.
24. Mira JP, Cariou A, Grall F, Delclaux C, Losser MR, Heshmati F, Cheval C, Monchi M, Teboul JL, Riche F, Leleu G, Arbibe L, Mignon A, Delpech M, Dhainaut JF.

Association of TNF2, a TNF-alpha promoter polymorphism, with septic shock susceptibility and mortality: a multicenter study. JAMA 1999;282:561-568.
25. Pociot F, Molvig J, Wogensen L, Worsaae H, Dalboge H, Baek L, Nerup J. A tumour necrosis factor beta gene polymorphism in relation to monokine secretion and insulin-dependent diabetes mellitus. Scand J Immunol 1991;33:37-49.
26. Bettinotti MP, Hartung K, Deicher H, Messer G, Keller E, Weiss EH, Albert ED. Polymorphism of the tumor necrosis factor beta gene in systemic lupus erythematosus: TNFB-MHC haplotypes. Immunogenetics 1993;37:449-454.
27. Badenhoop K, Schwarz G, Trowsdale J, Lewis V, Usadel KH, Gale EA, Bottazzo GF. TNF-alpha gene polymorphisms in type 1 (insulin-dependent) diabetes mellitus. Diabetologia. 1989;32:445-448.
28. Pociot F, Briant L, Jongeneel CV, Molvig J, Worsaae H, Abbal M, Thomsen M, Nerup J, Cambon-Thomsen A. Association of tumor necrosis factor (TNF) and class II major histocompatibility complex alleles with the secretion of TNF- alpha and TNF-beta by human mononuclear cells: a possible link to insulin- dependent diabetes mellitus. Eur J Immunol 1993;23:224-231.
29. Vinasco J, Beraun Y, Nieto A, Fraile A, Mataran L, Pareja E, Martin J. Polymorphism at the TNF loci in rheumatoid arthritis. Tissue Antigens 1997;49:74-78.
30. Majetschak M, Flohe S, Obertacke U, Schroder J, Staubach K, Nast KD, Schade FU, Stuber F. Relation of a TNF gene polymorphism to severe sepsis in trauma patients. Ann Surg 1999;230:207-214.
31. Boermeester MA, Van Leeuwen PA, Coyle SM, Wolbink GJ, Hack CE, Lowry SF. Interleukin-1 blockade attenuates mediator release and dysregulation of the hemostatic mechanism during human sepsis. Arch Surg 1995;130:739-748.
32. Pociot F, Molvig J, Wogensen L, Worsaae H, Nerup J. A TaqI polymorphism in the human interleukin-1 beta (IL-1 beta) gene correlates with IL-1 beta secretion in vitro. Eur J Clin Invest 1992;22:396-402.
33. Guasch JF, Bertina RM, Reitsma PH. Five novel intragenic dimorphisms in the human interleukin-1 genes combine to high informativity. Cytokine 1996;8:598-602.
34. Reinhart K, Wiegand-Lohnert C, Grimminger F, Kaul M, Withington S, Treacher D, Eckart J, Willatts S, Bouza C, Krausch D, Stockenhuber F, Eiselstein J, Daum L, Kempeni J. Assessment of the safety and efficacy of the monoclonal anti- tumor necrosis factor antibody-fragment, MAK 195F, in patients with sepsis and septic shock: a multicenter, randomized, placebo- controlled, dose- ranging study. Crit Care Med 1996;24:733-742.
35. Bowcock AM, Ray A, Erlich H, Sehgal PB. Rapid detection and sequencing of alleles in the 3' flanking region of the interleukin-6 gene. Nucleic Acids Res 1989;17:6855-6864.
36. Fugger L, Morling N, Bendtzen K, Ryder LP, Svejgaard A. BglII polymorphism in the human interleukin 6 (IL 6) gene. Nucleic Acids Res 1989;17:7548-7548.
37. Fugger L, Morling N, Bendtzen K, Ryder L, Odum N, Georgsen J, Svejgaard A. MspI polymorphism in the human interleukin 6 (IL 6) gene. Nucleic Acids Res 1989;17:4419-4419.
38. Fugger L, Morling N, Bendtzen K, Ryder L, Andersen V, Heilman C, Karup Pedersen F, Friis J, Halbert P, Svejgaard A. IL-6 gene polymorphism in rheumatoid arthritis, pauciarticular juvenile rheumatoid arthritis, systemic lupus erythematosus, and in healthy Danes. J Immunogenet 1989;16:461-465.
39. Bone RC. Sir Isaac Newton, sepsis, SIRS, and CARS. Crit Care Med 1996;24:1125-1128.

40. Tarlow JK, Blakemore AI, Lennard A, Solari R, Hughes HN, Steinkasserer A, Duff GW. Polymorphism in human IL-1 receptor antagonist gene intron 2 is caused by variable numbers of an 86-bp tandem repeat. Hum Genet 1993;91:403-404.
41. Danis VA, Millington M, Hyland VJ, Grennan D. Cytokine production by normal human monocytes: inter-subject variation and relationship to an IL-1 receptor antagonist (IL- 1Ra) gene polymorphism. Clin Exp Immunol 1995;99:303-310.
42. Blakemore AI, Tarlow JK, Cork MJ, Gordon C, Emery P, Duff GW. Interleukin-1 receptor antagonist gene polymorphism as a disease severity factor in systemic lupus erythematosus. Arthritis Rheum 1994;37:1380-1385.
43. Metcalfe KA, Hitman GA, Pociot F, Bergholdt R, Tuomilehto-Wolf E, Tuomilehto J, Viswanathan M, Ramachandran A, Nerup J. An association between type 1 diabetes and the interleukin-1 receptor type 1 gene. The DiMe Study Group. Childhood Diabetes in Finland. Hum Immunol 1996;51:41-48.
44. Fink MP, Payen D. The role of nitric oxide in sepsis and ARDS: synopsis of a roundtable conference held in Brussels on 18-20 March 1995. Intensive Care Med 1996;22:158-165.
45. Mathiak G, Szewczyk D, Abdullah F, Ovadia P, Rabinovici R. Platelet-activating factor (PAF) in experimental and clinical sepsis. Shock. 1997;7:391-404.
46. Buchman TG. Manipulation of stress gene expression: a novel therapy for the treatment of sepsis? [editorial; comment]. Crit Care Med 1994;22:901-903.
47. Spitzer JA. Cytokine stimulation of nitric oxide formation and differential regulation in hepatocytes and nonparenchymal cells of endotoxemic rats. Hepatology 1994;19:217-228.
48. Pfeilschifter J, Eberhardt W, Hummel R, Kunz D, Muhl H, Nitsch D, Pluss C, Walker G. Therapeutic strategies for the inhibition of inducible nitric oxide synthase--potential for a novel class of anti-inflammatory agents. Cell Biol Int 1996;20:51-58.
49. Meier J, Affeldt M, Opitz C, Kleber FX, Speer A. A common base change in the promoter region of the human endothelial NO- synthase (NOS3) gene. Hum Mutat 1996;8:394-394.
50. Milner CM, Campbell RD. Polymorphic analysis of the three MHC-linked HSP70 genes. Immunogenetics 1992;36:357-362.
51. Pociot F, Ronningen KS, Nerup J. Polymorphic analysis of the human MHC-linked heat shock protein 70 (HSP70-2) and HSP70-Hom genes in insulin-dependent diabetes mellitus (IDDM). Scand J Immunol 1993;38:491-495.
52. Janeway-CA J, Medzhitov R. Lipoproteins take their toll on the host. Curr Biol 1999;9:R879-R882.
53. Poltorak A, He X, Smirnova I, Liu MY, Huffel CV, Du X, Birdwell D, Alejos E, Silva M, Galanos C, Freudenberg M, Ricciardi CP, Layton B, Beutler B. Defective LPS signaling in C3H/HeJ and C57BL/10ScCr mice: mutations in Tlr4 gene. Science 1998;282:2085-2088.
54. Takeuchi O, Kawai T, Sanjo H, Copeland NG, Gilbert DJ, Jenkins NA, Takeda K, Akira S. TLR6: A novel member of an expanding toll-like receptor family. Gene 1999;231:59-65.
55. Schwandner R, Dziarski R, Wesche H, Rothe M, Kirschning CJ. Peptidoglycan- and lipoteichoic acid-induced cell activation is mediated by toll-like receptor 2. J Biol Chem 1999;274:17406-17409.
56. Yoshimura A, Lien E, Ingalls RR, Tuomanen E, Dziarski R, Golenbock D. Cutting edge: recognition of Gram-positive bacterial cell wall components by the innate immune system occurs via Toll-like receptor 2. J Immunol 1999;163:1-5

57. Takeuchi O, Kaufmann A, Grote K, Kawai T, Hoshino K, Morr M, Muhlradt PF, Akira S. Cutting edge: preferentially the R-stereoisomer of the mycoplasmal lipopeptide macrophage-activating lipopeptide-2 activates immune cells through a toll-like receptor 2- and MyD88-dependent signaling pathway. J Immunol 2000;164:554-557.
58. Poltorak A, Smirnova I, He X, Liu MY, Van-Huffel C, McNally O, Birdwell D, Alejos E, Silva M, Du X, Thompson P, Chan EK, Ledesma J, Roe B, Clifton S, Vogel SN, Beutler B. Genetic and physical mapping of the Lps locus: identification of the toll-4 receptor as a candidate gene in the critical region. Blood Cells Mol Dis 1998;24:340-355.
59. Takeuchi O, Hoshino K, Kawai T, Sanjo H, Takada H, Ogawa T, Takeda K, Akira S. Differential roles of TLR2 and TLR4 in recognition of gram-negative and gram-positive bacterial cell wall components. Immunity 1999;11:443-451.
60. Ohashi K, Burkart V, Flohe S, Kolb H. Cutting edge: heat shock protein 60 is a putative endogenous ligand of the toll-like receptor-4 complex. J Immunol 2000;164:558-561.
61. Cario E, Rosenberg IM, Brandwein SL, Beck PL, Reinecker HC, Podolsky DK. Lipopolysaccharide activates distinct signaling pathways in intestinal epithelial cell lines expressing Toll-like receptors. J Immunol 2000;164:966-972.

Chapter 7

CORTICOSTEROIDS IN SEPSIS

Sergey Goodman, M.D., Ph.D., Charles L. Sprung, M.D.
Hadassah Hebrew University Medical Center, Department of Anesthesiology and Critical Care Medicine, Jerusalem, Israel

Introduction

The use of corticosteroids in severe sepsis and septic shock has been controversial for decades. The present chapter will review the potential benefits and detriments of the use of corticosteroids in sepsis, the use of corticosteroids in animal models of sepsis and, with particular emphasis, their use in humans with severe sepsis and septic shock.

Beneficial and detrimental actions of Corticosteroids in sepsis

Corticosteroids act in many different ways. One of the most critical actions of steroids on the inflammatory process is their inhibitory effect on almost all known cytokines (1). It is believed that a prolonged and exaggerated release of these inflammatory mediators leads to organ dysfunction and steroids can reverse this process. The major component of the anti-inflammatory action of glucocorticoids may be their inhibition of the activity of nuclear factor kappa B (NF-$_{\kappa}$B) which activates the cytokine cascade (1). The inhibition is mediated via the induction of I$_{\kappa}$Bα inhibitory protein, which traps activated NF-$_{\kappa}$B in inactive cytoplasmic complexes (1). Corticosteroids may also suppress inflammation by increasing the synthesis of anti-inflammatory proteins, such as lipocortin 1, that have inhibitory effects on phospholipase A2, the rate-controlling enzyme governing the release of arachidonic acid from membrane phospholipids (2). In addition, steroids may inhibit the synthesis of inflammatory mediators through an inhibitory effect on enzyme induction such as the inhibition of the inducible cyclo-oxygenase 2 (COX-2), and by preventing the release of adhesion molecules such as ICAM-1 and VCAM-1 (3).

There are several mechanisms for the beneficial actions of corticosteroids in sepsis (Table I). The most physiologic benefit of corticosteroids would be replacement of the hormone in adrenal insufficiency. Unfortunately, most patients with severe sepsis and septic shock do not have adrenal insufficiency and many patients have elevated cortisol levels in sepsis (4). However, septic patients may have relative adrenal insufficiency (3). Corticosteroids may also act as vasodilators and improve cardiac function. Some studies have shown an improved cardiac output with steroids whereas others have not (5). Other metabolic effects of corticosteroids include increased glucagon secretion, liver protein synthesis and gluconeogenesis (6). Steroids stabilize cell and lysosomal membranes (7). Steroids have been shown to inhibit complement-induced granulocyte aggregation, disaggregate granulocytes and decrease endothelial cell damage by preventing oxygen-radical production (8). Corticosteroids also shift the oxyhemoglobin dissociation curve to the right, allowing an increased oxygen availability to the cells (9). Corticosteroids may also inhibit corticotropin-releasing factor (CRF) which regulates the release of adreno- corticotropic hormone (ACTH) and β-endorphin (10). The latter may depress cardiac function in shock. In fact, adreno-hypothalamopituitary interactions may be extremely important in the shock response. Corticosteroids restore the receptivity of catecholamine receptors (3). Glucocorticoids can prevent desensitization of α-adrenergic receptors and decrease the number of down regulated receptors (11). They may recouple catecholamine induced, desensitized adrenergic receptors and increase adrenergic receptor density in tissues (12).

Table 1. Beneficial Actions of Corticosteroids in Sepsis

Improve decreased adrenal function
Improve myocardial performance
Stimulate gluconeogenesis
Stabilize lysosomal and cell membranes
Inhibit complement-induced granulocyte aggregation and prevent oxygen radical mediated injury
Rightward shift in oxygen-hemoglobin dissociation curve
Interaction with endorphins
Enhance adrenergic receptivity

Despite the potential beneficial actions of corticosteroids, there are also detrimental effects, especially when steroids are given in high doses for long periods of time (Table 2) (6). In humans, complications have included superinfections, hyperglycemia, gastrointestinal bleeding, electrolyte disturbances, psychosis and arrhythmias (6).

Table 2. Detrimental Actions of Corticosteroids in Sepsis

Inhibit of neutrophilic bactericidal competency
Interfere with phagocytosis of antigens and subsequent intracellular digestion
Inhibition migration of cells to areas of inflammation
Large doses suppress cell-mediated hypersensitivity
Inhibit antigen processing by macrophages
Inhibit inflammatory response after antigen-antibody union

Corticosteroids in Animal Models

Although septic shock models in animals do not replicate the clinical situation (13), they do provide the rationale for the use of corticosteroids in patients. Many of these laboratory investigations suggested that prophylactic or early use of corticosteroids in sepsis and septic shock increased survival (14, 15). Hinshaw and his colleagues evaluated their use during challenge with live bacteria or endotoxin in dogs and baboons. In a baboon model of LD_{100} septic shock induced by the slow infusion of live organisms, corticosteroid (methylprednisolone 75 mg/kg over 12 hours) and antibiotic therapy initiated 30 minutes after bacteremia resulted in no deaths. When treatment was delayed by 120 minutes, 85% of the animals survived (16) and when it was begun 4 hours after the initial insult, overall survival decreased to 65% (17, 18). These data led to the belief that corticosteroids had to be given early, in high doses, and with appropriate antibiotic therapy for them to be beneficial.

Corticosteroids use in severe sepsis and septic shock in humans

The use of corticosteroids in patients with infections and sepsis has had its ups and downs. Corticosteroids were used first as anti-inflammatory agents in patients with infections even without the use of antibiotics (19). Later, steroids were used in combination with antibiotics (20). Corticosteroids were commonly used for patients with septic shock in the 1970s and early 1980s until two large prospective studies showed that they did not improve survival (21, 22). Since that time, steroids have not been commonly used in patients with severe sepsis and septic shock. However, over the last few years there has been a resurrection of the use of corticosteroids, secondary to recent studies showing a reversal of septic shock and potential improved survival with their administration (23, 24).

Weitzman and Berger (25) analyzed the design of 32 studies on the use of corticosteroids in patients with infections or sepsis published between 1950 and 1971. The criteria that they considered important in evaluating clinical studies were prospective design, concurrent controls, random allocation, double-blind technique, clear diagnostic criteria for entry and rating, stratification according to extent of disease, nature of underlying disease and observation of corticosteroid complications. The majority of studies they assessed had methodological flaws based on these criteria. They found greater non-compliance with proper study design in the 12 papers specifically dealing with septic shock. Due to their important paper, more recent studies of corticosteroids in patients with sepsis have had greater adherence to these methodological standards.

Kreger et al (26) showed in a retrospective study of Gram-negative bacteremia, that patients receiving corticosteroid therapy had a higher incidence of developing shock. They also demonstrated that patients treated with ≥ 4 gm/day of hydrocortisone for septic shock had a greater mortality than those patients not receiving steroids (72% compared to 36%, respectively). Schumer (27) reported a prospective study of the use of corticosteroids in septic shock in 1976. The definition of septic shock included a septic history, falling blood pressure and positive blood cultures. Treatment consisted of the intravenous administration of methylprednisolone (30 mg/kg), dexamethasone (3 mg/kg) or placebo at the time of diagnosis and repeated 4 hours later. Mortality was significantly lower in those patients treated with corticosteroids than placebo-treated patients (10% compared to 38%). Patients with a greater severity of shock had a greater mortality and the corticosteroid-treated patients did better than placebo treated patients at the different severities of shock. This was the first prospective, double-blind study clearly demonstrating a benefit in patients receiving steroids as adjunct therapy in septic shock and was the basis for the use of corticosteroids in these patients for many years thereafter. In 1984, Hoffman et al (28) demonstrated that dexamethasone (3 mg/kg) followed by a 1 mg/kg infusion every 6 hours for 48 hours reduced mortality from 56% to 10% in patients with severe typhoid fever compared to placebo. Patients were defined as having severe typhoid fever if they were febrile, had *S. typhi* or *S. parathyphi A.* cultured from the blood or bone marrow and abnormal state of consciousness or shock. The study was a randomized, double-blind, placebo controlled study. Interestingly, in this study, patients were treated with chloramphenicol and "standard" treatment did not include vasopressor or anti-arrhythmic agents, tracheal intubation or mechanical ventilation.

We performed a prospective, randomized, controlled study of corticosteroids in patients with septic shock (29). Septic shock was defined as a systolic blood pressure < 90 mmHg, evidence of decreased organ perfusion, bacteremia or an identified source of infection, and continued hypotension despite the administration of at least 500 ml of isotonic saline. At the time, many individuals were using corticosteroids based on Schumer's work (27). After speaking to Dr. Schumer, however, we were convinced that many of his patients were hypovolemic. The question in our study was whether corticosteroids could be efficacious in septic shock patients who were adequately volume repleted. Patients were randomized into methylprednisolone (30 mg/kg), dexamethasone (6 mg/kg) and control groups. Repeated doses of corticosteroids were given at 4 hours if shock persisted. Patients were treated late in shock (17 hours after the onset) and were in severe shock (average dopamine concentrations of more than 20 mcg/kg/min). Although ultimate in-hospital mortality and reversal of shock were not improved by corticosteroids (Figures 1 and 2), there were some short term improvements.

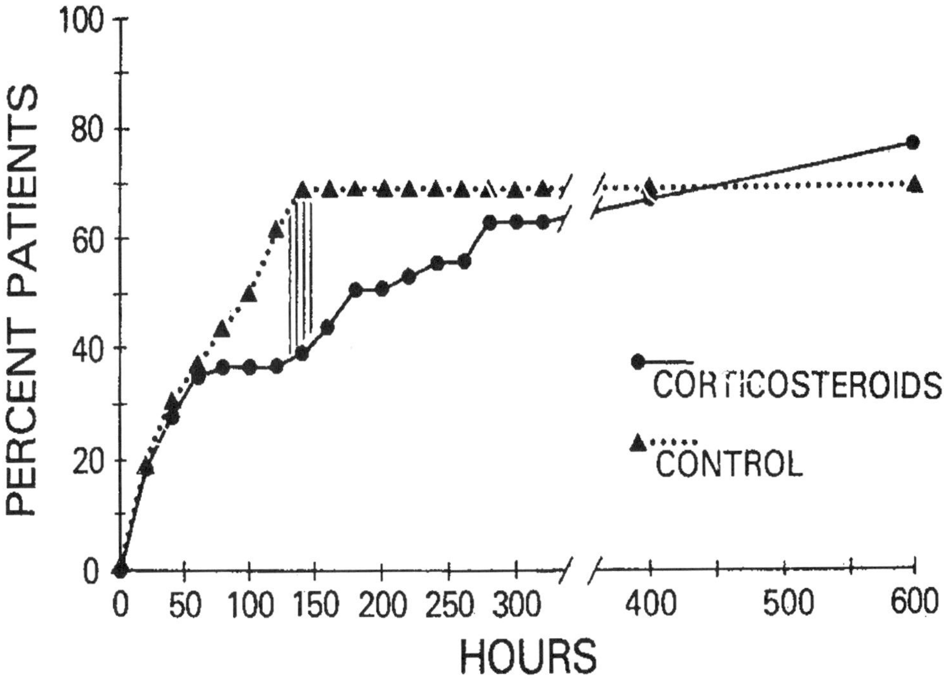

Figure 1. Hospital mortality in patients treated with corticosteroids and in control from the time of drug administration. From 133 to 150 hours after treatment the corticosteroids-treated group had improved survival ($p<0.05$, noted by shaded area) (29), reprinted with permission.

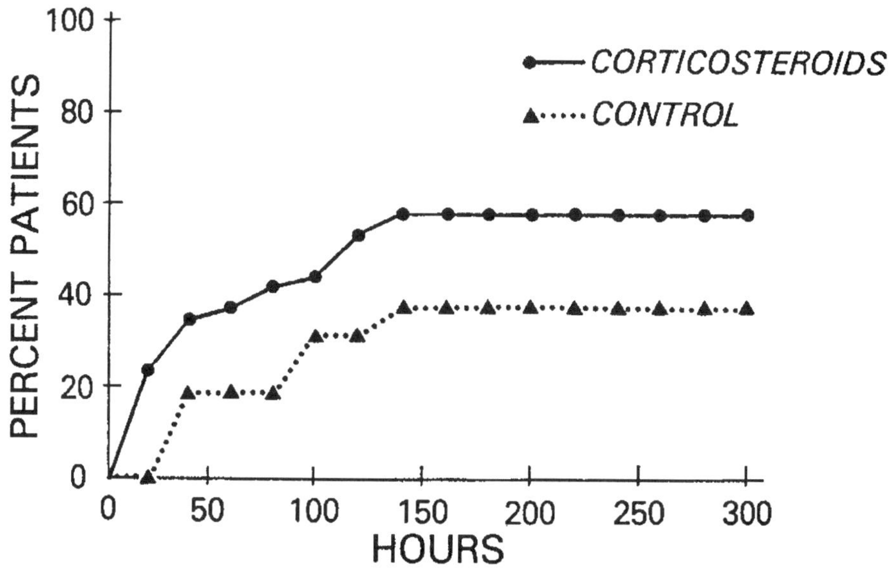

Figure 2. Reversal of shock in patients treated with corticosteroids and in controls from time of drug administration (29), reprinted with permission.

Corticosteroid-treated patients had a higher incidence of shock reversal at 24 hours, and those patients treated within 4 hours of shock with corticosteroids had a higher incidence of overall shock reversal. Furthermore, patients in the steroid groups had a lower mortality from 133-150 hours after the study drug administration. However, dexamethasone-treated patients had a higher incidence of superinfection. We speculated that further doses of corticosteroids after 4 hours could have resulted in continued reversal of shock after 24 hours and perhaps improved overall survival. During the 1980s, it was believed that extremely high doses of corticosteroids were required and that lack of efficacy in studies was related to the treatment of patients too late in the course of their sepsis. Therefore, two large multi-center prospective, randomized, double-blind, placebo-controlled studies of corticosteroids in patients treated early in sepsis were instituted (21, 22).

The Veterans Administration (VA) Systemic Sepsis Cooperative Study Group evaluated patients with sepsis (21). The definition of sepsis included a clinical suspicion of sepsis and at least 4 of the following 7 clinical signs within an 8-hour period: 1) fever or hypothermia, 2) tachycardia, 3) tachypnea, 4) hypotension, 5) abnormal while blood cell count, 6) thrombocytopenia, and 7) an invasive procedure during the preceding 48 hours or an obvious source of infection. In addition to antibiotics and intravenous fluids, patients received methylprednisolone (30 mg/kg) over 15 minutes followed by 5 mg/kg/hr infusion for 9 hours or placebo. Patients were treated within 2.8 hours of the diagnosis of sepsis. Because of issues of informed consent, all patients enrolled in the study had a normal mental status and had to sign their own informed consent. The 14-day mortality was not significantly different between the corticosteroid (21%) and placebo (22%) group (Figure 3).

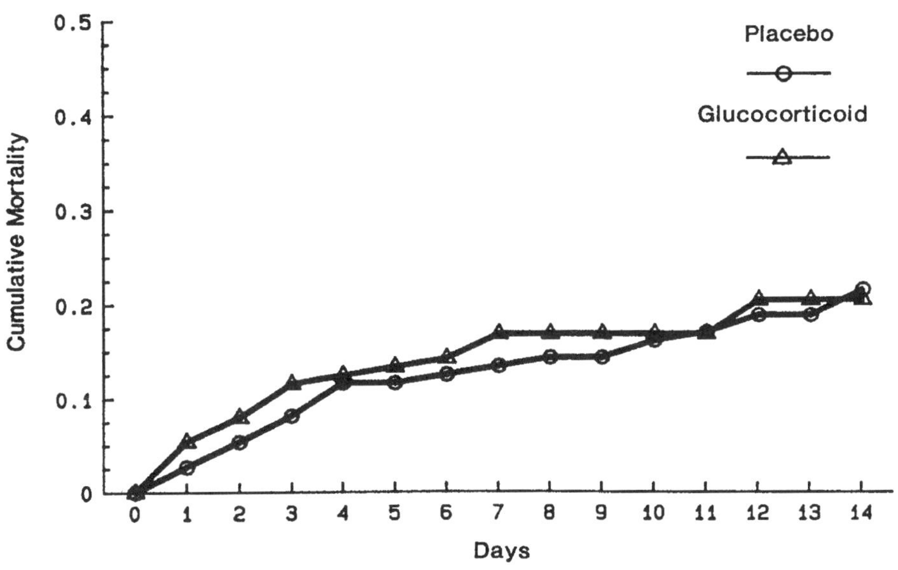

Figure 3. Cumulative mortality rates in all patients, according to treatment group (21), reprinted with permission.

Resolution of secondary infection was significantly higher in the placebo group than in the corticosteroid group ($p<0.05$), but mortality rates were similar for patients in both groups with unresolved infection.

The Methylprednisolone Severe Sepsis Study Group (22) evaluated patients with sepsis defined as: 1) clinical evidence of infection, 2) fever or hypothermia, 3) tachycardia, 4) tachypnea, and 5) the presence of at least one of the following manifestations of organ dysfunction – altered mentation, hypoxemia, elevated lactate or oliguria. Patients received standard therapies and methylprednisolone (30 mg/kg every 6 hours for a total of 4 doses) or placebo within 2 hours of the diagnosis of sepsis. The 14-day mortality tended to be higher in the methylprednisolone-treated patients (34%) compared to the placebo patients (25%) ($p=0.06$). In addition, corticosteroids did not prevent septic shock in those patients not in shock at study entry, nor did they reverse the shock of those patients already in septic shock Patients with renal dysfunction at study entry who received corticosteroids had a higher incidence of shock development and mortality ($p<0.05$). The incidence of secondary infection in the two groups did not differ but mortality directly attributed to secondary infection was higher in the steroid group than the placebo group ($p<0.05$) .

Two meta-analyses on the use of corticosteroids in sepsis were conducted subsequent to the above studies (30, 31). Lefering and Neugebauer (30) concluded that there was no overall beneficial effect of corticosteroids in patients with septic shock; there was some evidence (although not significant) for a positive effect in patients with Gram-negative sepsis. Gastrointestinal bleeding, secondary infections and hyperglycemia were not more frequent in patients treated with steroids (30). Cronin et al (31) concluded that current evidence provides no support for the use of corticosteroids in patients with sepsis or septic shock and suggests that their use may be harmful. Studies with the highest methodologic quality scores suggested a trend towards increased mortality overall (31). No difference in secondary infection rates was demonstrated but there was a trend towards increased mortality from secondary infections in patients receiving steroids (31). Studies of patients with sepsis receiving corticosteroids in high doses for short time periods have shown that steroids cannot prevent acute respiratory distress syndrome (ARDS) (32) or decrease mortality in patients with ARDS (33).

Despite this earlier disappointing clinical experience, in the last several years, the hypothesis that corticosteroids might be useful in septic shock has returned. Unlike previous hypotheses, the belief was that steroids might be useful to treat relative adrenal insufficiency or glucocorticoid resistance in target organs (34). In this case, much lower doses of corticosteroids used for longer periods of time than in previous studies have been speculated to be potentially useful.

In 1998, Bollaert et al (23), demonstrated in a prospective, randomized, double-blind, placebo-controlled study that patients treated with modest doses of hydrocortisone in the setting of pressor- dependent septic shock for more than 4 days resulted in a significant improvement in hemodynamics and a beneficial effect on survival. Septic shock was defined as an adaption to the ACCP/SCCM Consensus Conference criteria (35) and patients had to be receiving vasopressor therapy for more than 48 hours. Patients received hydrocortisone 100 mg intravenously 3 times daily for 5 days or matching placebo. Treatment was discontinued if the criteria of shock reversal were not fulfilled. If shock was reversed, treatment was continued with half doses for 3 days, quarter doses for 3 days and then stopped. Reversal of shock was defined by a stable systolic blood pressure > 90 mmHg for more than 24 hours without catecholamine or fluid infusions. Patients were in septic shock requiring catecholamines for 5 to 6 days. The hydrocortisone-treated patients had a higher incidence of 7-day shock reversal (68%) than the placebo-treated patients (21%) (p=0.007). At 28-day follow up, reversal of shock was higher in the hydrocortisone group (p=0.005) (Figure 4).

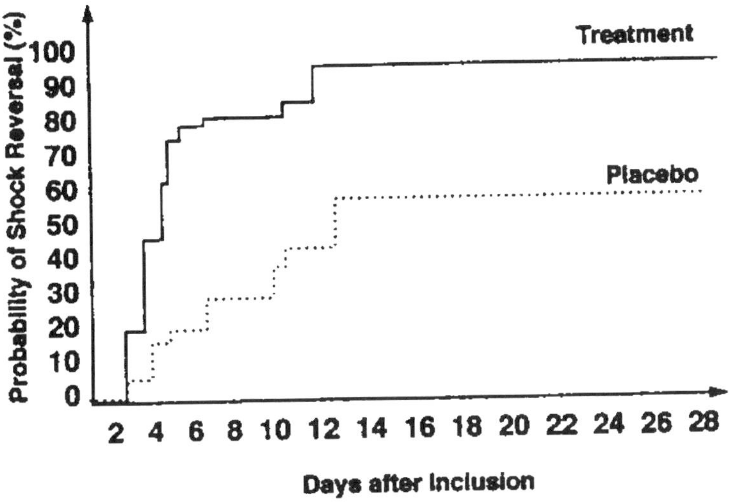

Figure 4. Kaplan-Meier estimates of 28-day reversal of shock (23), reprinted with permission.

The 28-day mortality was 32% in the hydrocortisone patients and 63% in the placebo patients (p=0.045) (Figure 5).

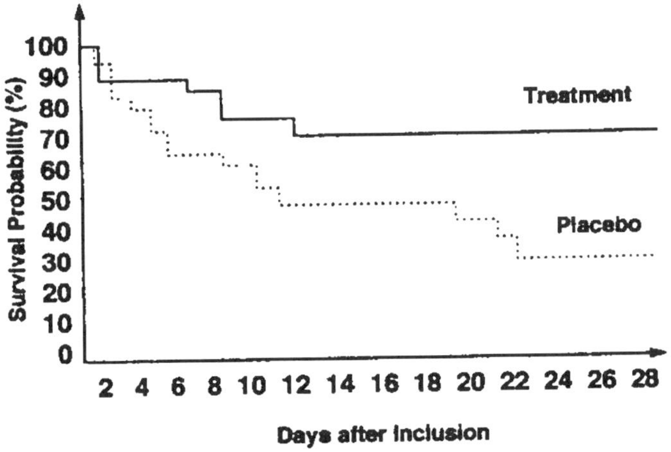

Figure 5. Kaplan-Meier estimates of 28-day all-cause mortality (23), reprinted with permission.

In 1999, Briegel et al (24) in a prospective, randomized, double- blind, single center study demonstrated that stress doses of hydrocortisone reduced the time to cessation of vasotherapy in septic shock. Septic shock was defined as the ACCP/SCCM Consensus Conference criteria and only those patients on vasopressor support with high cardiac output circulatory failure (cardiac index > 4.0 L/min/m^2) were randomized to the study groups. Patients were in septic shock for approximately 24 hours at the time of randomization. Patients were given 100 mg hydrocortisone over 30 minutes and followed by a continuous infusion of 0.18 mg/kg/hr or placebo. When septic shock was reversed, the dose of hydrocortisone was reduced to 0.08 mg/kg/hr. This dose was kept constant for 6 days. Hydrocortisone infusion was subsequently tapered in steps of 24 mg/day. Shock reversal was achieved in 18/20 patients treated with hydrocortisone vs. 16/20 patients treated with placebo. Hydrocortisone significantly reduced the time to cessation of vasopressor support. The median time of vasopressor support was 2 days in the hydrocortisone-treated group and 7 days in the placebo group (p=0.005). There were no differences in mortality (Figure 6).

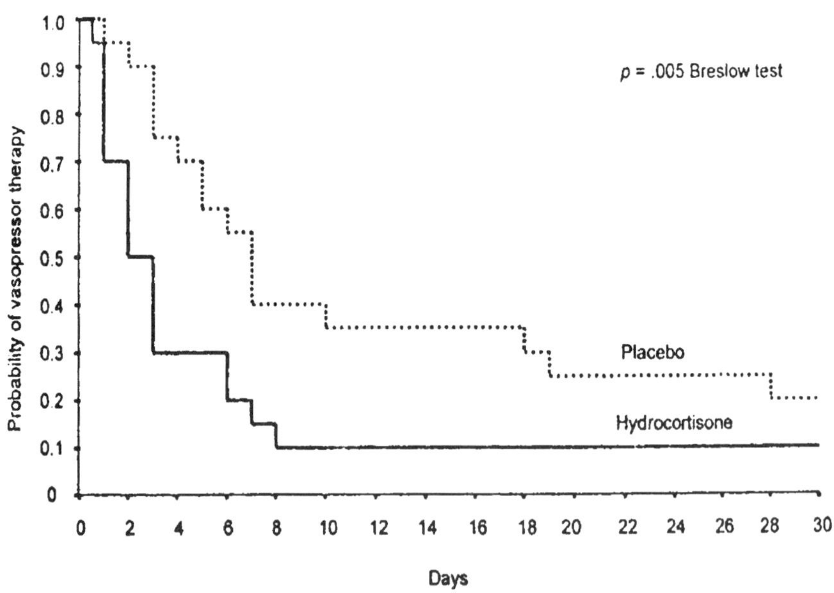

Figure 6. Kaplan-Meier curves demonstrating the probability of being on vasopressor therapy in the course of the study (24), reprinted with permission

A prospective, randomized, double-blind, placebo controlled trial of low doses of corticosteroids for longer periods in unresolving ARDS in 24 patients was associated with improvement in lung injury and reduced mortality (36).

From the aforementioned studies, extremely high pharmacologic doses of corticosteroids (30 mg/kg methylprednisolone) should not be used for adjunct therapy in patients with severe sepsis or septic shock. Lower doses of steroids (approximately 300-350 mg hydrocortisone a day) for longer periods of time (11-20 days) may be useful in reversing shock and decreasing mortality in patients with septic shock (23, 24). This may be especially true in patients receiving vasopressor agents for at least 24 hours and on appropriate antibiotic therapy. This therapy should be weighed carefully as physiologic doses of corticosteroids even for short periods may be associated with adverse effects (8). Infections may frequently develop in the absence of fever and must be pursued vigorously. In fact, in the study by Meduri et al. (36), weekly bilateral bronchoalveolar lavage was required for early detection of pneumonia.

REFERENCES

1. Auphan N. Immunosuppression by glucocorticoids: Inhibition of NF-$_{\kappa}$B activity through induction of I$_{\kappa}$B synthesis. Science 1995;270:286-290.
2. Chi EY, Henderson, WR, Klebanoff SJ: Phospholipase A_2-induced rat mast cell arachidonate metabolites. Lab Invest 1982; 47:579.
3. Carlet J. From mega to more reasonable doses of corticosteroids: A decade to recreate hope. Crit Care Med 1999; 27:672-674.
4. Schein RMH, Sprung CL, Marcial EH, Napolitano L, Chernow B. Plasma cortisol levels in patients with septic shock. Crit Care Med 1990;18:259-263.
5. Schein RMH, Long WM, Sprung CL. Controversies in management of sepsis and septic shock: Corticosteroids, naloxone, and nonsteroidal anti-inflammatory Agents. In: Sibbald WJ, Sprung CL, (editors). New Horizons - Perspectives on sepsis and septic shock. Fullerton: Society of Critical Care Medicine 1986; 339-368.
6. Melby JC. Systemic corticosteroid therapy: Pharmacology and endocrinologic considerations. Ann Intern Med 1974;81:505- 512.
7. Weismann G, Thomas L. Studies on lysosomes. 1. The effect of endotoxin tolerances and cortisone on the release of acid hydrolases from a granular fraction of rabbit liver. J Exp Med 1962;116:433-450.
8. Jacob HS, Craddock PR, Hammerschmidt DE et al. Complement-induced granulocyte aggregation: an unsuspected mechanism of disease. N Engl J Med 1980;302:780-784.
9. Kalter ES, Carlson RW, Thijs LG, et al. Effects of methylprednisolone on hemodynamics, arteriovenous oxygen difference, P_{50} and 2,3 DPG in bacterial shock. Crit Care Med 1982;10:662-666.
1. Vale W, Spiess J, Rivier C, Rivier J. Characterization of a 41 residue ovine hypothalamic peptide that stimulates secretion of corticotropin and β-endorphin. Science 1981;213:1394.

11. Barnes P. Beta-adrenergic receptors and their regulation. Am J Resp Crit Care Med 1995;152:838-860.
12. Davis AO, Lefkowitz RJ. Corticosteroid induced differential regulation of _-adrenergic receptors in circulating human polymorphonuclear leukocytes and mononuclear leukocytes. J Clin Endocrinol Metab 1980;51:599-605.
13. Eidelman LA, Sprung CL. Why have new effective therapies for sepsis not been developed? Crit Care Med 1994; 22:1330- 1334.
14. Greisman SE. Experimental gram-negative bacterial sepsis: Optimal methylprednisolone requirements for prevention of mortality not preventable by antibiotics alone. Proceed Soc Experiment Biol Med 1982;170:436-442.
15. Hellman A, Alestig K. High doses of corticosteroids in the treatment of septic shock. Acta Chir Scand Supp 1985;526:124- 128.
16. Hinshaw LB, Archer LT, Beller-Todd BK, et al. Survival of primates in lethal septic shock following delayed treatment with steroid. Circ Shock 1981;8:291-300.
17. Hinshaw LB, Beller-Todd BK, Archer LT. Effectiveness of steroid/antibiotic treatment in primates administered LD_{100} *Escherichia coli*. Ann Surg 1981;194:51-56.
18. Hinshaw LB, Beller-Todd BK, Archer LT. Current management of the septic shock patient: experimental basis for treatment. Circ Shock 1982; 9:543-553.
19. Kass EH. Finland M. Adrenocortical hormones and the management of infection. Ann Rev Med 1957;8:1-18.
20. Spink WW. ACTH and adrenocorticosteroids as therapeutic adjuncts in infectious diseases. N Engl J Med 1957;257:979-983.
21. Hinshaw L, Peduzzi P, Young E, Sprung C, Shatney C, et al. Effect of high-dose glucocorticoid therapy on mortality in patients with clinical signs of systemic sepsis. N Engl J Med 1987;317:659-665.
22. Bone RC, Fisher FJ, Clemmer TP, et al. A controlled trial of high-dose methylprednisolone in the treatment of severe sepsis and septic shock. N Engl J Med 1987;317:653-658.
23. Bollaert PE, Charpentier C, Levy B, Debouverie M, Audibert G, Larcan A. Reversal of late septic shock with supraphysiological doses of hydrocortisone. Crit Care Med 1998;26:645-650.
24. Briegel J, Forst H, Haller M, Schelling G, Kilger E, Kuprat G, Hemmer B, Hummel T, Lenhart A, Heyduck M, Stoll C, Peter K. Stress doses of hydrocortisone reverse hyperdynamic septic shock: A prospective randomized, double-blind, single-center study. Crit Care Med 1999;27:723-732.
25. Weitzman S, Berger S. Clinical trial design in studies of corticosteroids for bacterial infections. Ann Intern Med 1974;81:36-42.
26. Kreger BE, Craven DE, McCabe WR. Gram-negative bacteremia IV: re-evaluation of clinical features and treatment in 612 patients. Am J Med 1980;68:344-355.
27. Schumer W. Steroids in the treatment of clinical septic shock. Ann Surg 1976;184:333-341.
28. Hoffman SL, Punjabi NH, Kumulas S, et al. Reduction of mortality in chloramphenicol treated severe typhoid fever by high-dose dexamethasone. N Engl J Med 1984;310:82-88.
29. Sprung CL, Caralis PV, Marcial EH, Pierce M, Gelbard MA, Long WM, Duncan RC, Tendler MD, Karpf M. The effects of high-dose corticosteroids in patients with septic shock. N Engl J Med 1984;311:1137-1143.
30. Lefering R, Neugebauer EAM. Steroid controversy in sepsis and septic shock: A meta-analysis. Crit Care Med 1995;23:1294- 1303.

31. Cronin L, Cook DJ, Carlet J, Heyland DK, King D, Math B, Lansang MAD, Fisher CJ. Corticosteroid treatment for sepsis: A critical appraisal and meta-analysis of the literature. Crit Care Med 1995;23:1430-1439.
32. Luce JM, Montgomery AB, Marks JD, Turner J, Metz CA, Murray JF. Ineffectiveness of high-dose methylprednisolone in preventing parenchymal lung injury and improving mortality in patients with septic shock. Am Rev Respir Dis 1988;138:62-68.
33. Bernard GR, Luce JM, Sprung CL, Rinaldo JE, Tate RM, Sibbald WJ, Kariman K, Higgins S, Bradley R, Metz CA, Harris TR, Brigham K. High-dose corticosteroids in patients with the adult respiratory distress syndrome. N Engl J Med 1987;317:1565-1570.
34. Matot I, Sprung CL. Corticosteroids in septic shock: Resurrection of the last rites? Crit Care Med 1998;26:627-630.
35. American College of Chest Physicians/Society of Critical Care Medicine Consensus Conference Committee: American College of Chest Physicians/Society of Critical Care Medicine Consensus Conference. Definitions for Sepsis and organ failure and guidelines for the use of innovative therapies in sepsis. Crit Care Med 1992; 20:864-874.
36. Meduri GU, Headley S, Carson S, Umberger R, Kelso T, Tolley E. Prolonged methylprednisolone treatment improves lung function and outcome of unresolving ARDS. A randomized, double-blind, placebo-controlled trial. JAMA 1998;280:159-165.

Chapter 8

THE BIDIRECTIONAL EFFECT OF INFLAMMATION ON BACTERIAL GROWTH: A NEW INSIGHT INTO THE ROLE OF GLUCOCORTICOIDS IN THE RESOLUTION OF SEVERE INFECTIONS

G. Umberto Meduri, M.D.
Memphis Lung Research Program, Department of Medicine Divisions of Pulmonary and Critical Care Medicine and Infectious Disease & Department of Preventive Medicine, University of Tennessee, Memphis, and Veterans Affairs Medical Center, Memphis.

Supported by a grant from the Baptist Memorial Health Care Foundation and the Assisi Foundation of Memphis

Introduction

The ability to generate and respond to signaling molecules establishes a mechanism for regulated cell-to-cell communication. Cells coordinate their growth and proliferation with autocrine and paracrine signaling by means of low molecular weight polypeptides called cytokines. Innate or natural immunity is a highly conserved defense mechanism against infections found in all multicellular organisms (1). The inflammatory reaction is a fundamental component of the innate immune response, and its most proximal expression is characterized by the elaboration of proinflammatory cytokines—tumor necrosis factor (TNF)–α and interleukin (IL)–1β. Response to cytokines is generally viewed as exclusive to cells containing a defined nucleus, since cytokines are intended to work on well-defined eukaryotic cells with consequent signal transduction events.

When proinflammatory cytokines are present in optimal concentrations, they recruit both specific and nonspecific immune cells, nonlymphoid leukocytes (monocytes/macrophages, neutrophils, basophils, and eosinophils), and lymphocytes to the site of infection and activate them, thereby helping to eradicate the infection and restore homeostasis (2). However, there are occasions when the host defense response (HDR), in terms of inflammation, is exaggerated and protracted. In such cases, this primary defense process may instead cause enhanced tissue injury and maladaptive repair, leading to vital organ dysfunction and failure (3). Reduction in the effective concentration of proinflammatory mediators is an important component in the resolution of inflammation (4).

Glucocorticoids (GC) are a family of hormones produced by the adrenal cortex glands, which may be the most important physiological inhibitors of inflammation. A number of trials have demonstrated that patients with septic shock or ARDS do not benefit from a *short* course of massive doses of glucocorticoids administered early in the disease (5). However, a significant body of experimental literature has provided clear, although perhaps unappreciated, evidence that dosage and duration of GC administration influences treatment response and outcome in septic shock and in ARDS (6-17). Recently, four small double-blind, randomized trials evaluating prolonged GC therapy in patients with septic shock or unresolving ARDS (sepsis induced) have been completed (18-21). In all four, prolonged GC treatment was associated with a rapid, significant clinical improvement. In two of them, survival was an endpoint, and both reported a significant reduction in mortality (18,21). We have proposed that *duration* of glucocorticoid administration is a previously neglected critical variable in therapeutic outcome (22).

Endogenous and exogenous glucocorticoids exert most of their effects by activating ubiquitously distributed cytoplasmic heat shock protein-complexed glucocorticoid receptors (GR) with formation of the GC-GR complex (23). It is now appreciated that the GC-GR complex can modulate transcription in a *hormone-dependent manner* through interference with the activity of other transcription factors such as nuclear factor-κB (NF-κB) (24). NF-κB is a pleiotropic regulator, recognized as the critical transcription factor for the maximal expression of many genes central to the inflammatory response. GR-mediated transcriptional interference is achieved by four important mechanisms: (1) physically interacting with the p65 subunit with formation of an inactive (GR-NF-κB) complex (23), (2) inducing the inhibitory protein IκBα (23,25,26), (3) blocking degradation of IκBα via enhanced synthesis of IL-10 (27), and (4) by impairing TNF-α induced degradation of IκB α (28). Our group experience with prolonged glucocorticoid treatment in unresolving ARDS has led to a series of observations that have challenged the commonly accepted view of infections as amplifiers of inflammation in the activated host (29).

The concepts of microbial etiology and pathogenesis of infectious diseases have undergone revisions since the pioneer researcher of microbial diseases, Robert Koch, postulated the criteria for the microbial etiology of diseases. During the past decade, the emphasis in the study of the pathogenesis of infectious diseases has shifted from determining the function of the cellular players in the inflammatory response to the mediators which orchestrate this response (30). The relationship between bacteria and inflammation is traditionally viewed as unidirectional. Bacteria trigger inflammation, and inflammation—as part of the host innate immune response—destroys bacteria and localizes the spread of infection. Although correct, this simple relationship does not provide a complete picture of the pathogen-host interaction in acute life-threatening infections. This unchallenged (preconditioned) view of the pathogen-host interaction has influenced for years the interpretation of objective clinical data in critical care medicine. In the first part of this chapter, I will briefly review the clinical literature on nosocomial infections in acute respiratory distress syndrome (ARDS). Then I will present the results of a prospective study of ARDS patients that investigated longitudinally the relationship between circulatory and pulmonary proinflammatory cytokine levels, infections, and outcome. The findings of this study, as well as those of other groups, generated a novel hypothesis, suggesting that bacteria may grow in the presence of excessive cytokine levels. The second part of this chapter presents the results of recent *in vitro* studies in support of this new hypothesis.

Clinical observation in ARDS

ARDS is a frequent form of hypoxemic respiratory failure characterized by the acute development of diffuse lung inflammation. In mortality data, after day 3 of ARDS, most patients die following a prolonged period of ventilatory support, during which they often develop fever and other criteria for systemic inflammatory response syndrome (SIRS) (31), clinical manifestations of infection (32-34), and multiple organ dysfunction syndrome (MODS) (35,36). In the medical literature, sepsis is associated with fatality in 36% to 90% of ARDS nonsurvivors (32,33,35,36). At necropsy, 69% of ARDS nonsurvivors have histologic evidence of pneumonia (37). These observations led to the hypothesis that in ARDS a direct correlation may exist between development of nosocomial infections (NI), amplification of the systemic inflammatory response, and higher mortality (38). Faist and coworkers (39) proposed a two-hit hypothesis in which NIs represent a second insult to a previously injured and primed host, converting a low-grade or regulated host response into an accelerated or dysregulated host response (accelerated SIRS), triggering new or progressive organ dysfunction. Support for this hypothesis, however, relied only on clinical studies that did not use strict criteria for diagnosing NI. Furthermore, this broadly accepted pathophysiological hypothesis (second hit hypothesis) was never tested prospectively in ARDS.

NOSOCOMIAL INFECTIONS AND INFLAMMATION

Nosocomial infections and systemic inflammatory response in ARDS

We conducted a prospective study to investigate, at the onset of ARDS and during the progression of the disease, the longitudinal relationship between circulatory proinflammatory cytokine levels, infections, and outcome (29). In most patients, the etiology of ARDS was pulmonary or extrapulmonary sepsis. We reported that at the onset of ARDS, and over time, nonsurvivors (n = 17) had significantly ($p < 0.001$) higher plasma TNF–α, IL–1β, and IL–6 levels than survivors (n = 17) did (40). During the first week of ARDS, plasma cytokine levels declined in all survivors, whereas they remained persistently elevated in all nonsurvivors. Nosocomial infections were more frequent in patients with persistent cytokine elevation over time. The rate of nosocomial infection per day of mechanical ventilation was 1% in survivors and 8% in nonsurvivors. Moreover, none of the proven (n = 36) or suspected (n = 55) nosocomial infections caused either a transient or a sustained increase in plasma TNF–α, IL–1β, IL–6, and IL–8 levels above preinfection values (29). This latter finding is in agreement with the recent understanding of downregulation [also called lipopolysaccharide (LPS) tolerance] of an activated system (see discussion in reference 13). In these patients, a plasma IL-1β > 400 pg/ml on day 7 of ARDS was 100% accurate in predicting outcome (29). Sixty-seven percent of NI developed after day 10 of ARDS, and among nonsurvivors 15 of 18 nosocomial infections developed while plasma IL–1β was > 400 pg/ml. In addition to our work (29), two additional studies have described an association between high circulating IL–6 levels and increased rate of infections (41,42).

Ventilator-associated pneumonia and pulmonary inflammation in ARDS

The relationship between ventilator-associated pneumonia and pulmonary inflammation was evaluated in a series of prospective studies. We evaluated with bilateral bronchoalveolar lavage (BAL) 94 ARDS patients with 172 episodes of suspected ventilator-associated pneumonia (VAP) and compared BAL results from contralateral sites (43). Thirty-three of the 55 (60%) positive bronchoscopies had significant ($> 10^4$ CFU/ml) growth in only one side. Episodes with bilateral significant growth were more likely to be polymicrobial, to have a bacterial growth $> 10^5$ CFU/ml in the BAL, and to possess a higher percentage of polymorphonuclear (PMN) cells and intracellular microorganisms. These BAL findings indicated that episodes with a higher bacterial burden had cytological evidence of a more intense local inflammatory response and were more likely to be diffuse. Postmortem studies have also described a strong association between number of bacteria and severity of local inflammation (44-46). The traditional interpretation of these data would suggest that the more severe inflammation was the result of a higher bacterial burden; however, this relationship was challenged by the results of our prospective study (47).

In a longitudinal study of patients with ARDS subjected to bilateral BAL weekly and when clinical manifestations of VAP developed (47), we reported that at the onset of ARDS and over time, nonsurvivors had significantly ($p < 0.001$) higher BAL TNF–α, IL–1β, and IL–6 levels than survivors did (47). Nonsurvivors had a higher rate of ventilator–associated pneumonias than survivors (29). In 21 episodes of VAP, 16 unilateral and 5 bilateral pneumonia had excellent agreement between right and left BAL TNF–α, IL–1β, IL–6, total protein, and albumin levels. In other words, patients with unilateral pneumonia had similar TNF–α, IL–1β, and IL–6 levels in the BAL obtained from the lung with significant bacterial growth compared to the BAL from the contralateral lung without growth (29). Furthermore, VAPs were not associated with either a transient or a sustained increase in BAL TNF–α, IL–1β, IL–6, and IL–8 levels above preinfection values (29). In agreement with our results, the findings of a recent experimental study of gram-negative pneumonia indicated that persistent elevation in BAL proinflammatory cytokines is associated with failure to clear intrapulmonary bacteria despite a large influx of PMN in the airspaces (48).

Experimental and human studies have shown that a lung affected by ARDS is impaired in its ability to clear a bacterial challenge. Several intrinsic defects have been previously implicated, primarily those related to changes in the alveolar environment and the function of phagocytic cells (2). Polymorphonuclear cells recruited into the airspaces of patients with ARDS have shown evidence of impaired microbicidal activity (49,50); this mechanism partly explains the lung's inability to clear bacteria in spite of intense local inflammation. Furthermore, PMN clearing of bacteria is dose-dependent, and the efficiency of PMN bactericidal activity decreases with increasing bacterial load (51).

RECENT UNDERSTANDING OF BACTERIA AND CYTOKINE INTERACTION

In the interaction between a microorganism and its host, the host's defense does not go unchallenged (52). Several reports have shown that DNA viruses have the ability to interfere with extracellular cytokines or inhibit cytokine synthesis (52). Until recently, very little was known of the ability of bacteria to interfere with or to utilize extracellular cytokines secreted by the host cells or intracellular cytokines within phagocytic cells. Recent reports have shown that certain bacteria have receptors for cytokines IL-1β and TNF-α and that exposure of bacteria to these cytokines enhanced their growth (53-55).

Receptors

The surfaces of gram-negative bacteria have receptors for proinflammatory cytokines TNF–α and IL–1β (54-56), and the virulence property of the bacterium is altered as a consequence of cytokine binding (55). Porat et al. (53) reported that virulent strains of *E. coli* express receptors for IL–1β and demonstrated enhanced extracellular *in vitro* growth in the presence of biologically active recombinant IL–1β. Luo et al. (55) reported that TNF–α could bind efficiently to many strains of gram–negative bacteria and that TNF–α bacterium complexes can interact with TNF–α receptors present on eukaryotic cells. They also showed that TNF–α binding enhanced bacterial invasion of HeLa cells and phagocytosis by human and murine macrophages (55).

Enhanced bacterial growth with cytokines

Enhanced bacterial growth in the presence of cytokines has been reported for *E. coli,* IL–1β (53), interferon-gamma (57), IL–2, granulocyte macrophage colony stimulating factor (GM-CSF) (58), and *Staphylococcus aureus* (IL–4) (59). Two studies reported that the intracellular growth of *Mycobacterium avium-intracellular* complex was enhanced in human peripheral blood monocytes activated with the cytokines IL–3, IL–6, and GM-CSF (60,61).

Antiinflammatory cytokines have also been reported to promote bacterial growth. Two studies have shown that IL–10 and IL–4 can enhance the intracellular replication of bacteria. Park and Skerrett (62) reported that priming of human monocytes with IL–10 significantly enhanced the intracellular growth of *Legionella pneumophila.* Hultgren et al. (59) reported reduced growth of *S. aureus* in the joints of an IL-4–deficient mouse and showed that exposure of macrophages to IL–4 reduced intracellular killing of *S. aureus* without impairing phagocytosis.

NEW HYPOTHESIS AND HYPOTHESIS TESTING

The findings from our studies described above (29,40,47) suggested that final outcome in patients with ARDS is related to the magnitude and duration of the host inflammatory response, and that intercurrent nosocomial infections might be an epiphenomenon of prolonged intense inflammation. The increased rate of nosocomial infections might be explained by impaired host defense response. However, we hypothesized that cytokines secreted by the host during ARDS may indeed favor the growth of bacteria and explain the association between an exaggerated and protracted release of cytokines and the frequent development of nosocomial infections. To test this hypothesis, we conducted *in vitro* studies evaluating the extracellular and intracellular growth response of three clinically relevant bacteria in response to graded concentrations of proinflammatory cytokines TNF–α, IL–1β, and IL–6 (63,64). The bacteria used were fresh isolates of *Staphylococcus aureus*, *Pseudomonas aeruginosa,* and *Acinetobacter* sps. obtained from patients with ARDS. The bacteria were grown in 3 ml of RPMI/DMEM medium without serum or antibiotics. Intracellular growth was tested in human monocytic cell line U937 and in blood monocytes of normal healthy volunteers.

In these studies, we identified a U-shaped response of bacterial growth to proinflammatory cytokines. When the tested bacteria were exposed *in vitro* to a lower concentration (10 pg to 250 pg) of TNF–α, IL–1β, or IL–6—similar to the plasma values detected in ARDS survivors (40)—extracellular and intracellular bacterial growth was not promoted, and human monocytic cells were efficient in killing the ingested bacteria (63,64). On the contrary, when bacteria were exposed to higher concentrations of these of proinflammatory cytokines—similar to the plasma values detected in ARDS nonsurvivors (40)—intracellular and extracellular bacterial growth was enhanced in a dose-dependent manner (63,64). Blockade by specific neutralizing monoclonal antibodies (MoAb) significantly inhibited cytokine-induced extracellular and intracelullar bacterial growth (63,64).

The effects of cytokines on extracellular bacterial growth were seen only with fresh isolates and were lost after six *in vitro* passages (63). These findings indicate that, in the host milieu, *Staphylococcus aureus*, *Pseudomonas aeruginosa*, and *Acinetobacter* sps. may acquire a phenotypic ability to use cytokines as growth factors, and that subsequent removal of these pathogens from such milieu (after six *in vitro* passages) resulted in the loss of the acquired phenotype. This phenomenon of loss of responsiveness to cytokines was also recorded by Porat et al. (56).

The intracellular growth of *Staphylococcus aureus*, *Pseudomonas aeruginosa,* and *Acinetobacter* sps. was also tested after exposure of U937 monocytic cells to graded concentrations of lipopolysaccharide (LPS). At low priming concentrations of LPS, we observed a significant reduction in intracellular bacterial growth in comparison to control. However, at a priming concentration of LPS equal to or greater than 100 ng, all three bacterial isolates had a significant growth enhancement in comparison to control (all $p < 0.0001$, for all three bacteria). Taken together, our findings indicate that there may be a threshold of cellular activation at which phagocytic cells effectively kill ingested bacteria (Figure 1). Above this threshold of cellular activation, however, the intracellular micromilieu becomes favorable to the survival and replication of the ingested bacteria. It is likely that bacteria that are internalized, and under selective pressure, may adapt to an otherwise hostile microenvironment by switching on novel gene expression that enables them to utilize cytokines as their growth factors.

We then exposed U937 monocytic cells primed with the highest concentration of LPS (10 μg) to escalating concentrations (0 μg, 25 μg, 50 μg, 75 μg, 100 μg, 150 μg, and 250 μg) of methylprednisolone and quantified both intracellular bacterial growth and the intracellular transcription of TNF–α, IL–1β, and IL–6. We found that exposure of LPS-primed U937 monocytic cells to methylprednisolone prior to infection affected (in a dose-dependent manner) the mRNA expression of TNF–α, IL–1β, and IL–6, and the *in vitro* intracellular bacterial growth of internalized *Staphylococcus aureus*, *Pseudomonas aeruginosa,* and *Acinetobacter* sps (65).

The impairment in intracellular bacterial killing correlated with the increased expression of proinflammatory cytokines, while restoration of monocyte killing function upon exposure to methylprednisolone coincided with the downregulation of the expression of TNF–α, IL–1β, and IL–6. We found that, at the two highest concentrations of methylprednisolone (150 μg and 250 μg), the mRNA expression of all three cytokines was significantly blunted, irrespective of the LPS concentration. Hence, we presume that bacterial survival and replication within the phagocytic cells are functions of the cytokines expressed by such cells. In the presence of excessive activation, the intracellular environment appears to favor the emergence of new phenotypes of bacteria that are capable of utilizing cytokines for their growth. By showing that methylprednisolone can reduce (in a dose-dependent manner) the mRNA expression of TNF–α, IL–1β, and IL–6, and the intracellular bacterial growth of the tested bacteria, we provide experimental evidence to suggest a cause-and-effect relationship between excessive inflammation and bacterial growth.

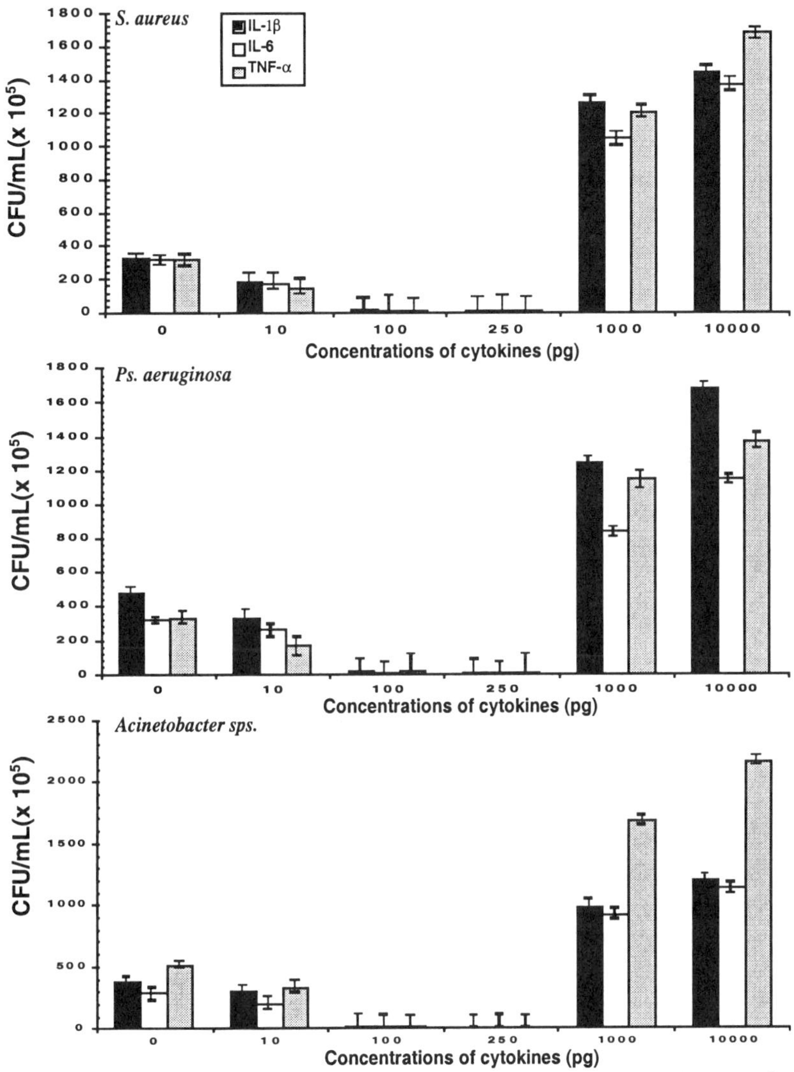

Figure 1. Intracellular bacterial growth of *S. aureus*, *P. aeruginosa,* and *Acinetobacter* sps. in U937 cells primed with graded concentrations of IL–1β, IL–6, and TNF–α. U937 cells (2 x 10^6) were primed with 0, 10, 100, 250 pg, and 1 and 10 ng of IL–1β, IL–6, and TNF–α. The primed cells were mixed with 6 x 10^6 CFU of each tested bacterium and incubated for 2 h. Extracellular bacteria were killed with gentamicin. The cells with internalized bacteria were incubated at 37°C for 12 h under an atmosphere of 5% CO_2. The cells were then lysed, serially diluted, and cultured onto Luria-Bertani (LB) agar (Difco, Detroit, Mich.) plates. The CFU per milliliter was estimated after 16 to 18 h of incubation. A concentration–dependent biphasic growth response was observed for all three bacteria, and this response was similar among the tested cytokines. The intracellular growth of three bacteria progressively decreased as the concentration of priming cytokines increased from 10 to 250 pg. However, this trend reversed when the priming concentration reached and

exceeded 1,000 pg, and intracellular bacterial growth increased manyfold ($P < 0.0001$, for all cytokines). Reproduced with permission from Kanangat.(40)

It is unclear how bacteria may use cytokines for their growth, since bacteria are prokaryotes without a defined nucleus and cytokines are intended to work on well-defined eukaryotic cells with consequent signal transduction events. However, in a host milieu, bacteria may adapt to eukaryotic cellular processes (66). Although, the subsequent sequence of intracellular events has not been delineated, it is possible that bacteria might use cytokines through receptor–mediated, signal-transduction-induced activities that would require the presence of biochemical processes akin to those seen in eukaryotic cells; cytokines may act on bacteria through a signaling process similar to that of eukaryotes, but involving different biochemical pathways; or bacteria may break down cytokines into biologically active fragments that are transported across the bacterial cell membranes and act on specific gene transcription and translation.

Conclusions

The bidirectional effects of proinflammatory cytokines on bacterial growth may help explain the frequent occurrence of nosocomial infections in patients with unresolving ARDS. Table 1 shows the traditional versus alternative interpretations of clinical findings in ARDS. If nosocomial infections in unresolving ARDS are indeed an epiphenomenon of exaggerated inflammation, it follows that treatment modalities that effectively decrease cytokine synthesis may reduce the incidence or severity of nosocomial infections.

Experimental evidence indicates that in patients with septic shock, excessive activation of the host defense response may induce noncompensated GC resistance in target organs, a condition potentially responsive to exogenous GC supplementation. Monocytes of patients with sepsis develop near-total GC resistance *in vitro* by adding cytokines (67). Nonsurvivors of septic shock have persistent immune cells activation of NF-κB, (68) and protracted elevation of circulating inflammatory cytokine levels over time (40,69-74).

We have recently hypothesized that if glucocorticoid inadequacy and/or resistance is an important pathophysiological component of *dysregulated* protracted systemic inflammation, then *prolonged* glucocorticoid therapy may be useful, not as an anti-inflammatory treatment *per se*, but as an hormonal supplementation to compensate for the host's inability to produce appropriately elevated levels of cortisol and/or for the inability of target organs to respond to endogenous cortisol (22). Within this hypothesis, we stated that adequate hormonal supplementation should modify the intracellular balance among activated transcription factors (NF-κB and GRα), thus converting an initially *dysregulated* (NF-κB-driven) expression of inflammatory genes into a *regulated* (GRα–driven) one, while concomitantly decreasing the HPA-axis release of ACTH and cortisol (22). In this context, glucocorticoid treatment is directed at the core pathogenetic mechanism of systemic inflammation in sepsis and ARDS, and should decrease (not suppress) the aberrant expression of inflammatory mediators.

Table 1. Traditional versus alternative interpretation of clinical data on nosocomial infections and inflammation in ARDS

Inflammation and bacteria
- Inflammation kills bacteria, vs
- Regulated inflammation kills bacteria while excessive (unregulated) inflammation may enhance bacterial growth

Nosocomial infections are more frequent
- In nonsurvivors, vs
- In patients with persistent cytokine elevation

Nosocomial infections
- Amplify inflammation (second hit hypothesis) and worsen MODS, vs
- Do not amplify inflammation (downregulation, or LPS tolerance)

The progression of systemic inflammation in ARDS
- Is amplified by nosocomial infections (≥ day 3 of ARDS), vs
- Is determined prior to day 3, by the success and/or failure of the host regulatory mechanisms

Glucocorticoid treatment in patients with unregulated systemic inflammation .
- Causes immunosuppression and enhances the risk for developing infections, vs
- If given in low doses for a prolonged period (≥ 7 days) may have an important immunomodulatory effect in regulating excessive inflammation and restoring homeostasis

For patients with sepsis or ARDS, there is no direct evidence yet demonstrating that GC treatment induces a reduction in intracellular activation of transcription factor NF-κB. Indirect evidence for such action, however, is provided by clinical studies that have monitored, before and during prolonged GC administration, the blood concentration of several mediators transcribed by NF-κB. In these studies, treatment was associated with a rapid, significant reduction in plasma levels of inflammatory mediators (TNF-α, IL-1β, IL-6, IL-8, PLA_2) (75,76) and adhesion molecules (77). So long as treatment was continued, the concentration of these biological markers continued to decrease, whereas physiological and clinical variables improved in parallel. In a randomized study of patients with sepsis-induced unresolving ARDS (21), this beneficial biological and physiological response was observed only in patients randomized to prolonged methylprednisolone administration, while no change was observed in those receiving placebo. In three clinical studies premature discontinuation of prolonged GC administration in septic shock (76) and in unresolving ARDS (78,79) was associated with physiological deterioration that improved with reinstitution of treatment. In the septic shock study, the clinical deterioration upon premature discontinuation of GC treatment was also accompanied by a rebound elevation of PLA_2, and C-reactive protein levels, which decreased with reinstitution of therapy (76). Finally, two reports provided indirect evidence to support the concept of endogenous GC resistance in patients with sepsis or unresolving ARDS. In a study of patients with septic shock, plasma cortisol levels decreased during hydrocortisone infusion and returned toward pre-treatment values after discontinuing therapy (76). Similarly, in patients with unresolving ARDS we have found that prolonged GC administration was associated with a significant reduction in ACTH and cortisol levels, in parallel with a reduction in circulating inflammatory cytokine levels (personal unpublished data).

No other treatment intervention in sepsis or ARDS has yet provided this level of evidence. Although, the results of four recent randomized studies are encouraging, pharmacokinetics and pharmacodynamics studies of exogenous GCs in sepsis and ARDS are not yet available to guide optimal drug administration, and today's treatment dosing is essentially empiric. Additional research is necessary to advance our understanding on the complex mechanisms that influence endogenous and exogenous GC activities at the cellular level during acute life-threatening inflammation.

REFERENCES

1. Suffredini AF, Fantuzzi G, Badolato R, Oppenheim JJ, O'Grady NP. New insights into the biology of the acute phase response. J Clin Immunol. 1999;19:203-214.
2. Meduri GU, Estes RJ. The pathogenesis of ventilator-associated pneumonia: II. The lower respiratory tract. Intensive Care Med. 1995;21:452-461.
3. Meduri GU. The role of the host defence response in the progression and outcome of ARDS: pathophysiological correlations and response to glucocorticoid treatment. Eur Respir J. 1996;9:2650-2670.
4. Rossi AG, Haslett C. Inflammation, cell injury, and apoptosis. In: Said SI, ed. *Proinflammatory and antiinflammatory peptides*. New York: Marcel Dekker, Inc.; 1998:9-24.
5. Jantz MA, Sahn SA. Corticosteroids in acute respiratory failure. Am J Respir Crit Care Med. 1999;160:1079-1100.

6. Levitin H, Kendrick MI, Kass EH. Effect of route of adminstration on protective action of corticosterone and cortisol against endotoxin. Proc Soc Exp Biol Med. 1956;93:306-309.
7. Weil MH, Allen KS. The effect of steroids on shock due to endotoxin. In: Mills LC, ed. *Inflammation and diseases of connective tissue; a Hahnemann symposium*. Philadelphia: Saunders; 1961:768-778.
8. Lillehei RC, Longerbeam JK, Bloch JH. Physiology and therapy of bacteremic shock. The American Journal of Cardiology. 1963:599-613.
9. Pitcairn M, Schuler J, Erve PR, Holtzman S, Schumer W. Glucocorticoid and antibiotic effect on experimental gram-negative bacteremic shock. Arch Surg. 1975;110:1012-1015.
10. Hinshaw LB, Coalson JJ, Benjamin BA, Archer LT, Beller BK, Kling OR, Hasser EM, Phillips RW. Escherichia coli shock in the baboon and the response to adrenocorticosteroid treatment. Surg Gynecol Obstet. 1978;147:545-557.
11. Hinshaw LB, Beller BK, Archer LT, Flournoy DJ, White GL, Phillips RW. Recovery from lethal Escherichia coli shock in dogs. Surg Gynecol Obstet. 1979;149:545-553.
12. Hinshaw LB, Archer LT, Beller-Todd BK, Coalson JJ, Flournoy DJ, Passey R, Benjamin B, White GL. Survival of primates in LD100 septic shock following steroid/antibiotic therapy. J Surg Res. 1980;28:151-170.
13. Greisman SE. Experimental Gram-negative bacterial sepsis: optimal methylprednisolone requirements for prevention of mortality not preventable by antibiotics alone. Proc Soc Exp Biol Med. 1982;170:436-442.
14. Jones RL, King G. The effects of methylprednisolone on oxygenation in experimental hypoxemic respiratory failure. J Trauma. 1975;15:297-303.
15. Hesterberg TW, Last JA. Ozone-induced acute pulmonary fibrosis in rats. Prevention of increased rates of collagen synthesis by methylprednisolone. Am Rev Respir Dis. 1981;123:47-52.
16. Hakkinen PJ, Schmoyer RL, Witschi HP. Potentiation of butylated-hydroxytoluene-induced acute lung damage by oxygen. Effects of prednisolone and indomethacin. Am Rev Respir Dis. 1983;128:648-651.
17. Kehrer JP, Klein-Szanto AJ, Sorensen EM, Pearlman R, Rosner MH. Enhanced acute lung damage following corticosteroid treatment. Am Rev Respir Dis. 1984;130:256-261.
18. Bollaert PE, Charpentier C, Levy B, Debouverie M, Audibert G, Larcan A. Reversal of late septic shock with supraphysiologic doses of hydrocortisone. Crit Care Med. 1998;26:645-650.
19. Briegel J, Haller M, Forst H, Schelling G, Kuprat G, Hemmer B, Peter K. Effect of hydrocortisone on reversal of hyperdynamic septic shock: A randomized, double-blind, placebo-controlled, single-center study. Shock. 1997;7:165.
20. Chawla K, Kupfer Y, Goldman I, Tessler S. Hydrocortisone reverses refractory septic shock. Crit Care Med. 1999;27:A33.
21. Meduri GU, Headley S, Carson S, Umberger R, Kelso T, Tolley E. Prolonged methylprednisolone treatment improves lung function and outcome of unresolving ARDS. A randomized, double-blind, placebo-controlled trial. JAMA. 1998;280:159-165.
22. Meduri GU. An historical review of glucocorticoid treatment in Sepsis. Disease pathophysiology and the design of treatment investigation. Sepsis. 1999;3:21-38.

23. Bamberger CM, Schulte HM, Chrousos GP. Molecular determinants of glucocorticoid receptor function and tissue sensitivity to glucocorticoids. Endocr Rev. 1996;17:245-261.
24. Didonato JA, Saatcioglu F, Karin M. Molecular mechanisms of immunosuppression and anti-inflammatory activities by glucocorticoids. Am J Respir Crit Care Med. 1996;154:S11-15.
25. Scheinman RI, Cogswell PC, Lofquist AK, Baldwin AS, Jr. Role of transcriptional activation of I kappa B alpha in mediation of immunosuppression by glucocorticoids. Science. 1995;270:283-286.
26. Wissink S, van Heerde EC, vand der Burg B, van der Saag PT. A dual mechanism mediates repression of NF-kappa B activity by glucocorticoids. Mol Endocrinol. 1998;12:355-363.
27. Wang P, Wu P, Siegel MI, Egan RW, Billah MM. Interleukin (IL)-10 inhibits nuclear factor kappa B (NF kappa B) activation in human monocytes. IL-10 and IL-4 suppress cytokine synthesis by different mechanisms. J Biol Chem. 1995;270:9558-9563.
28. Hofman TG, Hehner SP, Bacher S, Droge W, Schmitz ML. Various glucocorticoids differ in their ability to induce gene expression, apoptosis and to repress NF-kappaB-dependent transcription. FEBS Lett. 1998;441:441-446.
29. Headley AS, Tolley E, Meduri GU. Infections and the inflammatory response in acute respiratory distress syndrome. Chest. 1997;111:1306-1321.
30. Wilson M, Seymour R, Henderson B. Bacterial perturbation of cytokine networks. Infect Immun. 1998;66:2401-2409.
31. Bone RC, Balk RA, Cerra FB, Dellinger RP, Fein AM, Knaus WA, Schein RM, Sibbald WJ. Definitions for sepsis and organ failure and guidelines for the use of innovative therapies in sepsis. The ACCP/SCCM Consensus Conference Committee. American College of Chest Physicians/Society of Critical Care Medicine. Chest. 1992;101:1644-1655.
32. Montgomery AB, Stager MA, Carrico CJ, Hudson LD. Causes of mortality in patients with the adult respiratory distress syndrome. Am Rev Respir Dis. 1985;132:485-489.
33. Andrews CP, Coalson JJ, Smith JD, Johanson WG, Jr. Diagnosis of nosocomial bacterial pneumonia in acute, diffuse lung injury. Chest. 1981;80:254-258.
34. Seidenfeld JJ, Pohl DF, Bell RC, Harris GD, Johanson WG, Jr. Incidence, site, and outcome of infections in patients with the adult respiratory distress syndrome. Am Rev Respir Dis. 1986;134:12-16.
35. Bell RC, Coalson JJ, Smith JD, Johanson WG, Jr. Multiple organ system failure and infection in adult respiratory distress syndrome. Ann Intern Med. 1983;99:293-298.
36. Suchyta MR, Clemmer TP, Elliott CG, Orme JF, Jr., Weaver LK. The adult respiratory distress syndrome. A report of survival and modifying factors. Chest. 1992;101:1074-1079.
37. Meduri GU. Late adult respiratory distress syndrome. New Horiz. 1993;1:563-577.
38. Bone RC. Toward a theory regarding the pathogenesis of the systemic inflammatory response syndrome: what we do and do not know about cytokine regulation. Crit Care Med. 1996;24:163-172.
39. Faist E, Baue AE, Dittmer H, Heberer G. Multiple organ failure in polytrauma patients. J Trauma. 1983;23:775-787.
40. Meduri GU, Headley S, Kohler G, Stentz F, Tolley E, Umberger R, Leeper K. Persistent elevation of inflammatory cytokines predicts a poor outcome in ARDS. Plasma IL-1 beta and IL-6 levels are consistent and efficient predictors of outcome over time. Chest. 1995;107:1062-1073.

41. Romani L, Mencacci A, Cenci E, Spaccapelo R, Toniatti C, Puccetti P, Bistoni F, Poli V. Imparied neutrophil response and $CD4^+$ T helper cell development in interleukin 6-deficient mice infect with *Candida albicans*. J Exp Med. 1996;183:1345-1355.
42. Wagner HNJ, Bennett ILJ, Lasagna L, Cluff LE, Rosenthal MB, Mirick GS. The effect of hydrocortisone upon the course of pneumococcal pneumonia treated with penicillin. Bull Johns Hopkins Hosp. 1956;98:197-215.
43. Meduri GU, Reddy RC, Stanley T, El-Zeky F. Pneumonia in acute respiratory distress syndrome. A prospective evaluation of bilateral bronchoscopic sampling. Am J Respir Crit Care Med. 1998;158:870-875.
44. Rouby JJ, Martin De Lassale E, Poete P, Nicolas MH, Bodin L, Jarlier V, Le Charpentier Y, Grosset J, Viars P. Nosocomial bronchopneumonia in the critically ill. Histologic and bacteriologic aspects. Am Rev Respir Dis. 1992;146:1059-1066.
45. Johanson WG, Jr., Seidenfeld JJ, Gomez P, de los Santos R, Coalson JJ. Bacteriologic diagnosis of nosocomial pneumonia following prolonged mechanical ventilation. Am Rev Respir Dis. 1988;137:259-264.
46. Chastre J, Fagon JY, Bornet-Lecso M, Calvat S, Dombret MC, al Khani R, Basset F, Gibert C. Evaluation of bronchoscopic techniques for the diagnosis of nosocomial pneumonia. Am J Respir Crit Care Med. 1995;152:231-240.
47. Meduri GU, Kohler G, Headley S, Tolley E, Stentz F, Postlethwaite A. Inflammatory cytokines in the BAL of patients with ARDS. Persistent elevation over time predicts poor outcome. Chest. 1995;108:1303-1314.
48. Fox-Dewhurst R, Alberts MK, Kajikawa O, Caldwell E, Johnson MC, 2nd, Skerrett SJ, Goodman RB, Ruzinski JT, Wong VA, Chi EY, Martin TR. Pulmonary and systemic inflammatory responses in rabbits with gram- negative pneumonia. Am J Respir Crit Care Med. 1997;155:2030-2040.
49. Martin TR, Pistorese BP, Hudson LD, Maunder RJ. The function of lung and blood neutrophils in patients with the adult respiratory distress syndrome. Implications for the pathogenesis of lung infections. Am Rev Respir Dis. 1991;144:254-262.
50. Chollet-Martin S, Jourdain B, Gibert C, Elbim C, Chastre J, Gougerot-Pocidalo MA. Interactions between neutrophils and cytokines in blood and alveolar spaces during ARDS. Am J Respir Crit Care Med. 1996;154:594-601.
51. Clawson CC, Repine JE. Quantitation of maximal bactericidal capability in human neutrophils. J Lab Clin Med. 1976;88:316-327.
52. Kotwal GJ. Microorganisms and their interaction with the immune system. J Leukoc Biol. 1997;62:415-429.
53. Porat R, Clark BD, Wolff SM, Dinarello CA. Enhancement of growth of virulent strains of *Escherichia coli* by interleukin-1. Science. 1991;254:430-432.
54. Zav'yalov VP, Chernovskaya TV, Navolotskaya EV, Karlyshev AV, MacIntyre S, Vasiliev AM, Abramov VM. Specific high affinity binding of human interleukin 1 beta by Caf1A usher protein of Yersinia pestis. FEBS Lett. 1995;371:65-68.
55. Luo G, Niesel DW, Shaban RA, Grimm EA, Klimpel GR. Tumor necrosis factor alpha binding to bacteria: evidence for a high-affinity receptor and alteration of bacterial virulence properties. Infect Immun. 1993;61:830-835.
56. Porat RB, Clark D, Wolf SM, Dinarello CA. IL-1b and Escherichia coli. Science. 1992;258:1562-1563.
57. Hogan JS, Todhunter DA, Smith KL, Schoenberger PS, Sordillo LM. Growth responses of coliform bacteria to recombinant bovine cytokines. J Dairy Sci. 1993;76:978-982.

58. Denis M, Campbell D, Gregg EO. Interleukin-2 and granulocyte-macrophage colony-stimulating factor stimulate growth of a virulent strain of *Escherichia coli*. Infect Immun. 1991;59:1853-1856.
59. Hultgren O, Kopf M, Tarkowski A. Staphylococcus aureus-induced septic arthritis and septic death is decreased in IL-4-deficient mice: role of IL-4 as promoter for bacterial growth. J Immunol. 1998;160:5082-5087.
60. Denis M, Gregg EO. Recombinant tumour necrosis factor-alpha decreases whereas recombinant interleukin-6 increases growth of a virulent strain of *Mycobacterium avium* in human macrophages. Immunology. 1990;71:139-141.
61. Shiratsuchi H, Johnson JL, Ellner JJ. Bidirectional effects of cytokines on the growth of *Mycobacterium avium* within human monocytes. J Immunol. 1991;146:3165-3170.
62. Park DR, Skerrett SJ. IL-10 enhances the growth of *Legionella pneumophila* in human mononuclear phagocytes and reverses the protective effect of IFN-γ: differential responses of blood monocytes and alveolar macrophages. J Immunol. 1996;157:2528-2538.
63. Meduri GU, Kanangat S, Stefan J, Tolley E, Schaberg S. Cytokines Iβ-1β, IL-6, and TNF-α enhance *in vitro* growth of bacteria. Am J Respir Crit Care Med. 1999;161:961-967.
64. Kanangat S, Meduri GU, Tolley EA, Patterson DR, Meduri CU, Pak C, Griffin JP, Bronze MS, Schaberg DR. Effects of cytokines and endotoxin on the intracellular growth of bacteria. Infect Immun. 1999;67:2834-2840.
65. Meduri GU, Kanangat S, Tolley E, Patterson D, Meduri CU, Bronze MS, Schaberg D. Effects of glucocorticoids on the intracellular growth of bacteria in lipopolysaccharide-primed human monocytic cells [abstract]. In: *First International Congress on Cytokines/Chemokines in Infectious Diseases*. Bethesda, MD: American Association of Immunologists; 1999:131.
66. Falkow S. Perspectives series: host/pathogen interactions. Invasion and intracellular sorting of bacteria: searching for bacterial genes expressed during host/pathogen interactions. J Clin Invest. 1997;100:239-243.
67. Molijn GJ, Spek JJ, van Uffelen JC, de Jong FH, Brinkmann AO, Bruining HA, Lamberts SW, Koper JW. Differential adaptation of glucocorticoid sensitivity of peripheral blood mononuclear leukocytes in patients with sepsis or septic shock. J Clin Endocrinol Metab. 1995;80:1799-1803.
68. Bohrer H, Qiu F, Zimmermann T, Zhang Y, Jllmer T, Mannel D, Bottiger BW, Stern DM, Waldherr R, Saeger HD, Ziegler R, Bierhaus A, Martin E, Nawroth PP. Role of NF kappa B in the mortality of sepsis. J Clin Invest. 1997;100:972-985.
69. Damas P, Ledoux D, Nys M, Vrindts Y, De Groote D, Franchimont P, Lamy M. Cytokine serum level during severe sepsis in human IL-6 as a marker of severity. Ann Surg. 1992;215:356-362.
70. Calandra T, Gerain J, Heumann D, Baumgartner JD, Glauser MP. High circulating levels of interleukin-6 in patients with septic shock: evolution during sepsis, prognostic value, and interplay with other cytokines. The Swiss-Dutch J5 Immunoglobulin Study Group. Am J Med. 1991;91:23-29.
71. Calandra T, Baumgartner JD, Grau GE, Wu MM, Lambert PH, Schellekens J, Verhoef J, Glauser MP. Prognostic values of tumor necrosis factor/cachectin, interleukin-1, interferon-alpha, and interferon-gamma in the serum of patients with septic shock. Swiss-Dutch J5 Immunoglobulin Study Group. J Infect Dis. 1990;161:982-987.

72. Pinsky MR, Vincent JL, Deviere J, Alegre M, Kahn RJ, Dupont E. Serum cytokine levels in human septic shock. Relation to multiple- system organ failure and mortality. Chest. 1993;103:565-575.
73. Sullivan JS, Kilpatrick L, Costarino AT, Jr., Lee SC, Harris MC. Correlation of plasma cytokine elevations with mortality rate in children with sepsis. J Pediatr. 1992;120:510-515.
74. Dofferhoff AS, de Jong HJ, Bom VJ, van der Meer J, Limburg PC, de Vries-Hospers HG, Marrink J, Mulder PO, Weits J. Complement activation and the production of inflammatory mediators during the treatment of severe sepsis in humans. Scand J Infect Dis. 1992;24:197-204.
75. Meduri GU, Headley S, Tolley E, Shelby M, Stentz F, Postlethwaite A. Plasma and BAL cytokine response to corticosteroid rescue treatment in late ARDS. Chest. 1995;108:1315-1325.
76. Briegel J, Kellermann W, Forst H, Haller M, Bittl M, Hoffmann GE, Buchler M, Uhl W, Peter K. Low-dose hydrocortisone infusion attenuates the systemic inflammatory response syndrome. The Phospholipase A2 Study Group. Clin Investig. 1994;72:782-787.
77. Golden E, John B, Stentz F, Tolley EA, Meduri GU. Interleukin-8 and Soluble Intercellular adhesion molecule-1 during acute respiratory distress syndrome and in response to prolonged methylprednisolone treatment (Abstract). Shock. 2000;13:42S
78. Ashbaugh DG, Maier RV. Idiopathic pulmonary fibrosis in adult respiratory distress syndrome. Diagnosis and treatment. Arch Surg. 1985;120:530-535.
79. Hooper RG, Kearl RA. Established ARDS treated with a sustained course of adrenocortical steroids. Chest. 1990;97:138-143.

Chapter 9

ANTI-INFLAMMATORY THERAPY IN SEPSIS

Jonathan Sevransky, M.D. and Charles Natanson, M.D.
Johns Hopkins University and the National Institutes of Health

Introduction

Despite advances in supportive care and medical technology, the mortality rate from sepsis remains high (35-50%) (1). It is the most common cause of death in non-cardiac intensive care units, and the incidence appears to be rising (2). Over the last 20 years, prevailing thought has attributed much of the morbidity and mortality of sepsis to an overexuberant host inflammatory response to bacteria or bacterial products. In preclinical studies, agents designed to limit this host pro-inflammatory response showed promising effects, prompting numerous clinical trials.

Two approaches have been taken to limit this host inflammatory response. The first involved the use of agents to directly limit the production or biologic effects of pro-inflammatory mediators. The second used agents to neutralize the ability of bacterial products in the bloodstream to elicit a host pro-inflammatory response (Figure 1). The first approach used glucocorticoids at high doses administered at the onset of sepsis to inhibit inflammation. This proved unsuccessful. More recently, glucocorticoids in lower doses administered later in the course of sepsis have been studied. Several small studies in select groups of patients suggest a beneficial role for this treatment. In the last 15 years with advances in biology, therapies targeted against specific pro-inflammatory mediators (such as tumor necrosis factor α, interleukin-1, etc) have been developed. These agents, similar to glucocorticoids, inhibit inflammation but more selectively target specific mediators. Individual trials of these mediator-specific anti-inflammatory agents did not prove successful. However, when examined as a group, the trials suggest a small beneficial treatment effect, indicating that the hypothesis linking excessive production of pro-inflammatory mediators with the morbidity and mortality of sepsis has merit. It is not yet clear why the more marked beneficial effects seen in animal studies of anti-inflammatory agents have not been duplicated in clinical trials.

The second approach to limiting an overexuberant host response to infection involved the use of anti-endotoxin therapies. In contrast to the glucocorticoid and mediator specific anti-inflammatory therapies, this strategy targets bacterial products in the circulation with the expectation that neutralizing these bacterial toxins will limit the host pro-inflammatory response and thereby improve outcome (Figure 1). Approximately one dozen clinical trials of anti-endotoxin therapies in patients with sepsis or at high risk for sepsis have been performed. These trials do not show consistent beneficial effects in patients with sepsis. In the following pages we will summarize these clinical trials targeting the host inflammatory response in sepsis, and describe some of the preclinical studies that lead to these sepsis trials.

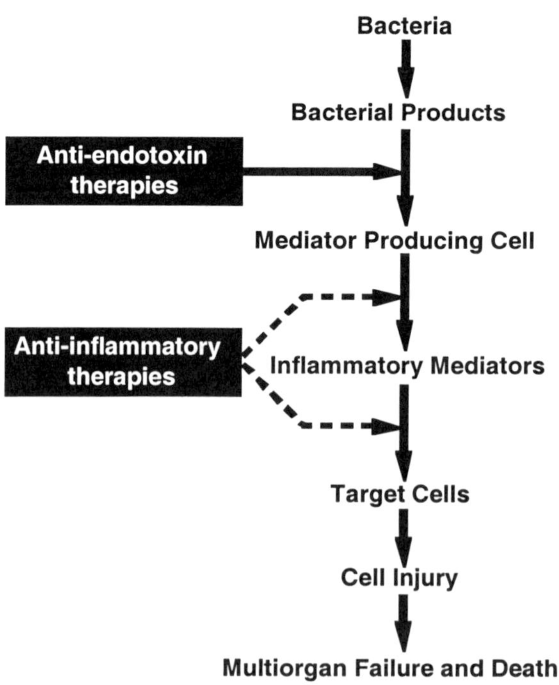

Figure 1. Different mechanisms of action for anti-endotoxin and anti-inflammatory therapies

Glucocorticoids in sepsis

Experiments suggesting a role for glucocorticoid therapy in sepsis were first performed in the 1930s. In adrenalectomized animals, glucocorticoid replacement lead to improved survival rates (3). Patients with meningococcemia were also shown to develop adrenal hemorrhage and shock, suggesting a role for adrenal replacement therapy (4). Further, bacteria and bacterial products such as endotoxin were found to incite a potent inflammatory response, and in animals, steroid therapy, either with or without antibiotics could limit this proinflammatory response and improve survival (5-10). These studies lead to clinical trials investigating the use of short courses of high dose glucocorticoid therapy in patients with sepsis or at risk for sepsis. Unfortunately, these trials did not show consistent beneficial effects with the use of glucocorticoids in sepsis and septic shock (11-18) (Figure 2).

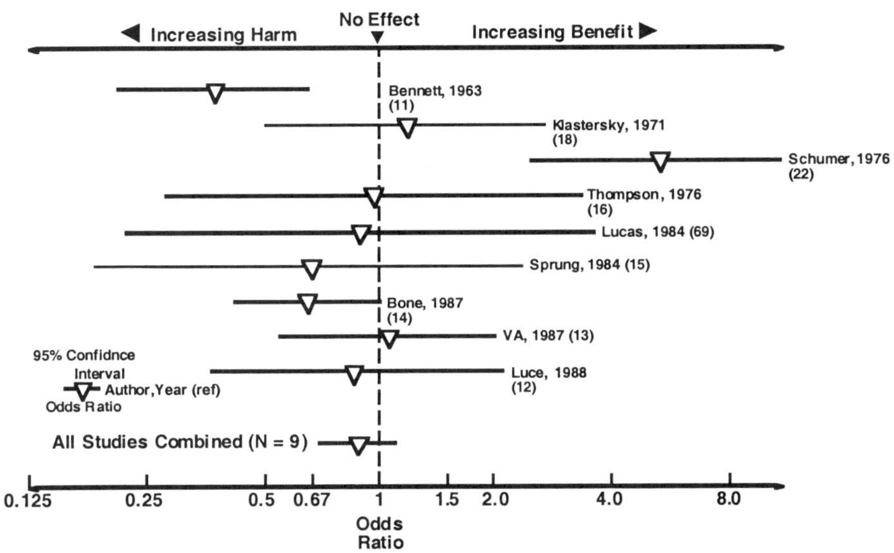

Figure 2. Survival odds ratios and 95% confidence intervals in nine clinical trials of high-dose corticosteroids in patients with sepsis and septic shock. Modified with permission from 21.

To better understand the results of these clinical trials, we and others have performed meta-analyses of the individual trials (19-21). These meta-analyses all confirmed the lack of benefit with this approach seen in the individual clinical trials. Of note, one study by Schumer et al. (22) demonstrated a beneficial treatment effect that was significantly different (p=0.001) from the other studies included in the meta-analysis. If this outlier is excluded from the meta-analysis, high dose glucocorticoid therapy was actually significantly harmful in patients with septic shock [Odds ratio (OR) 0.70; 95% confidence interval (CI) 0.546 to 0.913; p=0.001). This harmful effect could be explained in part by the fact that in some trials (14, 23), glucocorticoids induced immunosuppression and patients treated with glucocorticoids had higher rates of secondary infections. Given the lack of efficacy seen in these studies and potential harm, the use of high dose short-term glucocorticoids as an adjunctive therapy in patients with sepsis is no longer recommended (19-21).

Some recent reports have suggested that glucocorticoids given in a different manner may have a role in a subset of patients with sepsis. Several studies have suggested that patients with sepsis may have an inadequate hypothalamic-pituitary-adrenal axis and that this leads to decreased survival. It is not clear whether this ineffective axis is caused by relative decreases in production of glucocorticoids or the inability of target tissues to respond adequately to glucocorticoids (24). These observations have prompted studies to examine whether physiologic "stress dose" steroids may be effective in the treatment of sepsis.

Bollaert et al studied 41 patients with septic shock who required vasopressor support for greater than 48 hours to either hydrocortisone or placebo in addition to standard therapy (25). Prior to enrolling patients in the study, a short corticotrophin stimulation test was performed to exclude frank adrenocortical insufficiency (defined by an absolute plasma cortisol concentration >18 ug/dL). The primary endpoint was reversal of shock; the secondary endpoint was 28 day mortality rates. The patients receiving hydrocortisone showed a trend towards improved survival ($p=0.09$). In addition, patients randomized to hydrocortisone therapy were significantly more likely to be weaned from vasopressor support at 7 and 28 days ($p < 0.005$, both).

Two additional studies support these findings. Breigel et al studied patients with hyperdynamic septic shock (26). Patients with a cardiac index greater than 4 L/min who had been in shock for under 72h were randomized to either hydrocortisone (100 mg IV bolus followed by an infusion of 0.18/mg/kg/h) or placebo. There was no significant difference in mortality rates between the placebo and hydrocortisone treated patients. However, patients treated with hydrocortisone were weaned off vasopressor support significantly faster than patients randomized to placebo ($p=0.005$). Chalwa et al also studied low dose glucocorticoid therapy in patients with persistent vasopressor requirements (27). Patients in shock for greater than 72h were randomized to either hydrocortisone 100 mg every eight hours or placebo. Patients randomized to hydrocortisone were significantly more likely to recover from shock than were placebo treated individuals. There was however no significant difference in mortality.

Despite the small size of these 3 trials (i.e. 41 patients in one and 40 each of the other two), all showed a significant reduction in the amount and duration of vasopressor agents required (25-27). None of these three studies however, possibly related to their small sample sites, showed a significant improvement in survival rates with glucocorticoid treatment. The difference between these recent trials and the earlier multi-center trials relates to the patients selected, and the dosing and timing of administration of the glucocorticoid therapy. In the earlier studies, glucocorticoids were given at supraphysiologic doses early after the diagnosis of sepsis in an attempt to counter the overexuberant inflammatory response. In addition, these doses were given for only a brief period of time, in most cases under 72h. In contrast, the recent trials enrolled only patients with refractory pressor dependent shock, later in the course of the syndrome and continued glucocorticoid therapy for longer periods of time. The doses given in the recent studies were between 5 and 30 times less than the doses used in the previous studies. The entrance criteria for the studies using short-term high dose glucocorticoid therapy included patients on vasopressors as well as patients that never received vasopressors.

Mediator- Specific Anti-inflammatory Therapy in Sepsis

In the last two decades with advances in biotechnology a number of specific pro-inflammatory mediators have been described which are involved in the pathophysiology of the sepsis syndrome. The proinflammatory mediator thought primarily responsible and therefore most implicated was tumor necrosis factor-α (TNF-α). There have been nine published trials of monoclonal antibodies to TNF-α, enrolling over 4000 patients. In addition, three published trials used soluble tumor necrosis factor receptors (sTNFr) to limit the effects of circulating TNF-α. Three studies of Interleuken-1 receptor antagonists (IL-Lra) enrolled approximately 1900 patients. Three studies used ibuprofen for prostaglandin inhibition in sepsis. Further there were two trials of bradykinin antagonists and two trials of platelet activating factor antagonists. In total six types of mediator specific anti-inflammatory agents enrolled more than 10,000 patients.

Anti-TNF therapies

There is strong scientific rational to identify TNF-α as one of the primary mediators of the sepsis syndrome. Endotoxin challenged normal volunteers develop elevated levels of serum tumor necrosis factor along with tachycardia, tachypnea and falls in blood pressure, all of which are seen in patients with sepsis (28). In animal models of sepsis TNF-α challenges have been demonstrated to reproduce most of the cardiovascular derangements seen in sepsis. Similarly, in meningococcal infections, serum tumor necrosis factor levels have been demonstrated to correlate with mortality rates. Furthermore, pre-treatment with therapies to inhibit tumor necrosis factor have been shown to improve survival rates in animal models of sepsis.

These preclinical studies formed the basis for clinical trials of agents that inhibit TNF-α in patients with the sepsis syndrome.

Nine clinical trials using monoclonal antibodies against TNF-α (TNF-MAb) have been published. Five of these trials were double-blinded in design (21, 29-32), while four were open label studies (33-36). The double-blinded studies were, on average, larger than the open-label studies. None of the nine trials showed a significant improvement in survival rates. The mortality rate in the control groups ranged from 32% to 60%, with an average mortality of 42%. However, the treatment effects of the anti-TNF MAb were similar across the nine studies (p=0.87). If these nine studies of monoclonal antibodies against TNF-α are analyzed together, there is a small non-significant trend towards improved survival rates in the patients treated with anti-TNF MAb therapy (OR 1.10; 95% CI 0.97 to 1.25 p=0.14).

Soluble tumor necrosis factor receptors have also been tested in human clinical trials. Soluble TNF receptors (sTNFr) are shed from cells in the circulation and can be produced in large quantities by biologic engineering techniques. These receptors bind to circulating TNF, and lower its bioavailability. Three double-blinded clinical trials have been published, enrolling in total approximately 2000 patients (32, 37, 38). None of the individual trials showed a significant reduction in mortality rates for treated patients. One of the trials showed that high doses of high molecular weight p80 sTNFr significantly increased mortality rate (39). In two trials using the low molecular weight p55 sTNFr at much lower doses than in the higher molecular weight group, there was a small non-significant effect similar to anti-TNF MAb. However, as studied in clinical trials, neither of these agents designed to limit the biological effects of TNF-α in the circulation significantly improved mortality rates.

Interleukin-1 receptor antagonists

Interleukin-1 is another pro-inflammatory cytokine that when administered to humans or animals can reproduce many of the manifestations of the sepsis syndrome. Interleukin-1 receptor antagonist (IL-1ra) is a protein produced by macrophages, which binds to interleukin receptors, thus limiting the biologic activity of interleukin-1. These IL-1 inhibitors were given in three clinical trials in patients with sepsis and septic shock. One small trial was open-labeled, enrolling 99 patients (40). Two larger trials, enrolling 696 and 893 patients respectively were double-blinded (41, 42). Although the open-label trial suggested a large treatment effect for Il-1ra, the phase III double-blind studies did not confirm this large treatment effect (41, 42). None of the studies showed a significant improvement in survival rates. When the three studies are analyzed together, there was a small, non-significant improvement in survival rate, with a control mortality rate of 36% and a treated mortality rate of 31% (OR 1.18; 95% CI 0.97 to 1.44; p=0.10), similar to that seen with the TNF MAb trials.

Clinical trials of other mediator specific anti-inflammatory therapies

Platelet activating factor, a phospholipid has been suggested to promote the release of cytokines in sepsis as well as the development of the acute respiratory distress syndrome, (a frequent sequelae of the sepsis syndrome). Two double-blind studies have explored the use of platelet- activating factor receptor antagonists (PAFra) (43, 44). These studies were notable for having a high control mortality rate (50%); however, treatment with PAFra still showed only a small beneficial treatment effect that was not statistically significant (OR 1.20; 95% CI 0.92 to 1.57).

Bradykinin can stimulate the release of pro-inflammatory cytokines such as TNF and IL-1 and has been shown to promote vasodilatation and increase vascular permeability. Two double-blinded studies have examined the use of bradykinin antagonists in patients with the sepsis syndrome (45, 46). Neither study showed a significant improvement in survival rates. Even when the studies are analyzed together, there was no significant effect on survival rates of those bradykinin antagonists (OR 0.91; 95% CI 0.65 to 1.27).

Endotoxin has been shown to increase prostaglandin synthesis, which can in turn cause increased airway resistance, hypoxemia, pulmonary hypertension, tachycardia, and hypotension in animal models of sepsis (47, 48). Ibuprofen, a prostaglandin inhibitor, has been shown in animal models of sepsis to reverse these cardiopulmonary effects (47, 48). Three double-blinded studies have explored the use of ibuprofen in patients with sepsis (46, 49, 50). None of these studies showed a significant effect on mortality rates. When examined as a group, the control mortality rate was 40% and the treatment mortality rate was 37%, suggesting again a small, non significant improvement in survival rates (OR 1.22; 95% CI 0.78 to 1.58 p=0.14).

To date no individual trial of a mediator specific anti-inflammatory agent has significantly improved mortality rates. Further, when the individual trials are grouped into classes of agent such as anti-TNF MAb or IL-1ra, none of these classes of agents showed a significant improvement in mortality (51). However, when all of these classes of agents are examined together as a meta-analysis, an approach taken adapted from several previous papers (21, 51, 52), several trends become obvious. The mortality rates across control treated groups for each class of agent were remarkably similar, ranging from 35-50%. This consistency suggests that the trials were studying patients with similar severity of illness, and that the standard therapies for the sepsis syndrome (i.e. cardiovascular support and antibiotic therapy) were administered with similar results. Most trials did show a similar small non-significant reduction in mortality in the treated groups. When all these studies are pooled in a meta-analysis, a significant treatment effect is seen (See Fig 3). The mortality rate in treated patients was 36 percent, while in the control group the mortality rate was 39%. This demonstrates an absolute reduction in mortality of 3%, and a 7.5 % decreased relative risk of mortality. In effect, a trial of an anti-inflammatory agent with a similar treatment effect may need to enroll up to 6000 patients to show statistical significance for such a small treatment effect (52). This small treatment effect may explain why none of the previously published studies have shown a statistically significant improvement in mortality.

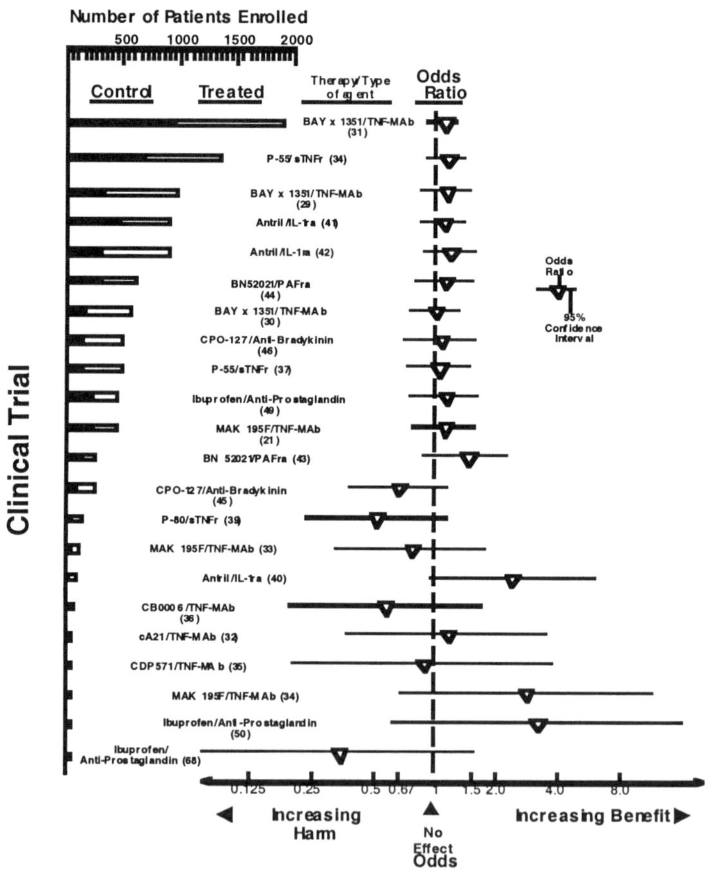

Figure 3. Survival odds ratio and 95% confidence intervals in 22 clinical trials of non-glucocorticoid anti-inflammatory agents ranked by size of clinical trial. TNF-Mab, tumor necrosis factor monoclonal antibody; IL-ra, interleuken receptor antagonist; PAFra, platelet-activating factor receptor antagonist; sTNFr, soluble tumor necrosis factor receptor antagonist. Modified with permission (21).

Thus these mediator specific anti-inflammatory agents appear to have small beneficial treatment effects. These small treatment effects bolster the hypothesis that the sepsis syndrome derives, at least in part, from an overexuberant host inflammatory response. However, it is not clear why the treatment effects in human clinical trials were so small compared with the large treatment effects seen in preclinical studies. Possible causes for this treatment difference may include differences in timing of administration, in patient population, and in selection of patients. In addition, it is possible that the severity of infection, or type and location of infection may play a role. A better understanding of why these clinical trials have failed as well as the difference between septic human and animals models of sepsis may help researchers develop new anti-inflammatory therapies or make better use of current therapies.

Anti-endotoxin therapy in sepsis

Endotoxin, a lipopolysaccaride present on the outer cell wall of gram-negative bacteria, has been offered as a key mediator in the development of the sepsis syndrome and septic shock. Endotoxin is composed of two antigens, a highly conserved lipid –A moiety, which appears to cause many of the toxic effects of the molecule, and an O- side chain. Infusion of endotoxin into experimental animals and normal human volunteers can reproduce many of the hemodynamic manifestations of the sepsis syndrome (53, 54). Some have hypothesized that endotoxin may be important not only in patients with gram-negative sepsis but in those with gram-positive sepsis also. In such patients, inadequate perfusion of the gut mucosa during gram-positive infection could allow endotoxin from gut flora to enter the systemic circulation, and thereby worsen the cardiovascular abnormalities. Thus endotoxin might be a therapeutic target not only in patients with gram-negative infections, but possibly in all types of shock associated with inadequate gut perfusion. The first studies of anti-endotoxin agents used antiserum or polyclonal antibodies directed at common epitopes among gram-negative bacteria. Later studies employed monoclonal antibodies.

We have previously examined the results of 10 clinical trials of anti-endotoxin therapies in sepsis both as a group, and as a meta-analysis (21, 55). Seven of these studies examined therapeutic treatment with anti-endotoxin therapy (56-62); three of the studies examined prophylactic treatment in high risk populations (58, 63, 64). When the 2605 patients enrolled in all 10 studies are analyzed as a group, treatment with these agents did not have a significant beneficial effect (OR 1.1; 95% CI 0.932 to 1.32 $p=0.24$). When the 7 therapeutic trials are examined, there was a trend towards benefit for treatment with anti-endotoxin agents that did not reach statistical significance. If the seven studies are however examined for consistency, two studies were significant outliers (p=0.04) (56, 57). These two studies by Ziegler et al demonstrated a beneficial effect (OR 1.98; 95% CI; 1.32 to 3.005; p=0.001) that was significantly different (p=0.001) from the lack of beneficial effect seen in the other five studies (OR 0.5; 95% CI O.428 to 0.526; p=0.84).

In summary, most of the trials using antibodies and anti-serum against endotoxin have not shown a consistent beneficial effect in patients with sepsis (65). Of concern, there are *in vitro* experiments that show that the agents used in human clinical trials do not adequately bind or neutralize endotoxin. (66). It is not clear whether the lack of efficacy of these anti-endotoxin therapies results from failure of the agents to have necessary biologic effect or from failure of the hypothesis that endotoxin should be a therapeutic target in sepsis. Recent trials have attempted to address this issue. Preliminary data (published only in press releases) suggest that the use of proteins derived from neutrophil granules that bind to endotoxin have not shown benefit in hemorrhagic shock. Small trials using hemoperfusion with polymyxin B-immobilized fibers suggest that hemoperfusion may lower endotoxin levels, but large-scale trials have not been performed to assess outcomes (67).

Conclusion

Preclinical studies have suggested that an overexuberant inflammatory response may be responsible for the morbidity and mortality associated with sepsis. In animal models of sepsis two successful approaches were studied to limit this inflammatory response. The first involved blocking the effects of host pro-inflammatory mediators. Glucocorticoids and mediator-specific anti-inflammatory agents were successful in animal models in improving outcome from sepsis. However, in clinical trials, use of high doses of glucocorticoids early in sepsis did not improve outcome. Some of the clinical studies with high dose glucocorticoids noted an increased risk of superinfection. Lower doses of glucocorticoids may be helpful later, in vasopressor dependent patients with sepsis. None of the individual trials of mediator specific anti-inflammatory agents showed significant benefit. Of note, in one trial, higher doses of sTNFr actually increased mortality rates in patients with sepsis (39). However, when the 22 published trials are examined as a whole, there appears to be some small benefit to this approach. It appears possible though that high doses of either glucocorticoid therapy or sTNFr are harmful in specific populations of patients with sepsis.

It is not yet clear why the large benefits seen in animal studies of anti-inflammatory agents have not been replicated in human clinical trials.

The second approach to limiting the inflammatory response involves blocking the effects of bacterial products on the host immune response. Again, despite favorable preclinical studies, the use of anti-endotoxin agents has not been shown to have a significant beneficial effect in human clinical trials. It is unclear whether this failure is related to a lack of necessary biologic effects of the agents tested or whether this is an improper approach. Further studies of more effective anti-endotoxin strategies are warranted.

REFERENCES

1. Wheeler, AP, and GR. Bernard. Treating patients with severe sepsis. N Eng J Med 1999;340:207-214.
2. Linde-Swirbe, WT, DC. Angus, J. Carcillo, et al. Age specific incidence and outcome of sepsis in the US. Crit Care Med 1999;27:A33.
3. Hartman, F. A., and W. J. M. Scott. Protection of adrenalectomized animals against bacterial intoxication by an extract of the adrenal cortex. J Exp Med 1932;55:63-69.
4. Sacks, M. S. Fulminating septicemia associated with purpura and bilateral adrenal hemorrhage (Waterhouse-Friderichsen Syndrome); report of two cases with review of the literature. Ann Int Med 1936:1105-1114.
5. Hinshaw, L. B., L. T. Archer, and B. K. Beller-Todd. Survival of primates in LD100 septic shock following steroid/antibiotic therapy. J Surg Res 1980;28:151-170.
6. Fabian, T. C., and R. Patterson. Steroid therapy in septic shock. Survival study in a laboratory model. Am Surgeon 1982;48:614-617.
7. Hinshaw, L. B., B. K. Beller-Todd, L. T. Archer, et al. Effectiveness of steroid antibiotic treatment in primates administered LD100 Eschericia coli. Ann Surg 1981;194:51-56.
8. Hinshaw, L. B., D. J. Flournoy, L. T. Archer, et al. Recovery from lethal Escherichia coli shock. Surg Gyn Ob 1979;149:545-553.
9. White, G. L., L. T. Archer, B. K. Beller-Todd, et al. Increased survival with methylprednisolone treatment in canine endotoxin shock. J Surg Res 1978;25.
10. Beller-Todd, B. K., L. T. Archer, R. Passey, et al. Effectiveness of modified steroid-antibiotic therapies for lethal sepsis in the dog. Arch Surg 1983;118:1293-1299.
11. Bennett, I. L., M. Finland, M. Hamborger, et al. The effectiveness of hydrocortisone in the management of severe infection. JAMA 1963;183:462-465.
12. Luce, J. M., A. B. Montgomery, J. D. Marks, et al. Ineffectiveness of high-dose methylprednisolone in preventing parenchymal lung injury and improving mortality in patients with septic shock. Am Rev Respir Dis 1988;138:62-68.
13. The Veterans Administration Systemic Sepsis Cooperative Study Group. Effect of high-dose glucocorticoid therapy on mortality in patients with clinical signs of systemic sepsis. N Engl J Med 1987;317:653-658.

14. Bone, R., C. Fisher, T. Clemmer, et al. A controlled trial of high dose methylprednisolone in the treatment of severe sepsis and septic shock. N Engl J Med 1987;317:653-8.
15. Sprung, C., P. Caralis, E. Marcial, et al. The effects of high dose corticosteroids in patients with septic shock. N Eng J Med 1984;311:1137-43.
16. Thompson, W. L., H. T. Gurley, B. A. Lutz, et al. Inefficacy of glucocorticoids in shock (double-blind study). Clin Res 1976;24:258A.
17. Schumer, W. Steroids in the treatment of clinical shock. Ann Surg 1976;184:133-139.
18. Klastersky, J., R. Cappell, and L. Debusscher. Effectiveness of betamethasone in management of severe infections. N Eng J Med 1971;284:1248-1250.
19. Cronin, L., D. J. Cook, and J. Carlet. Corticosteroid treatment for sepsis: a critical appraisal and meta-analysis of the literature. Crit Care Med 1997;23:1430-1439.
20. Lefering, R., and E. A. Neugebauer. Steroid controversy in sepsis and septic shock: a meta-analysis. Crit Care Med 1995;23:1294-1303.
21. Zeni, F., B. Freeman, and C. Natanson. Anti-inflammatory therapies to treat sepsis and septic shock: a reassessment. Crit Care Med 1997;25:1095-1100.
22. Schumer, W. Steroid in the treament of clinical septic shock. Arch Surg 1976;184: 537-541.
23. The Veterans Association Systemic Sepsis Cooperative Study Group. Effect of high dose glucocorticoid therapy on mortality in patients with clinical signs of sepsis. N Engl J Med 1987;317:653-658.
24. Meduri, G., and G. Chrousos. Duration of glucocorticoid treatment and outcome in sepsis. Chest 1998;114:355-359.
25. Bollaert, P.-E., C. Charpentier, B. Levy, et al. Reversal of late septic shock in with supraphysiologic doses of hydrocortisone. Crit Care Med 1998;26:645-650.
26. Briegel, J., H. Forst, M. Hallar, et al. Stress doses of hydrocortisone reverse hyperdynamic septic shock: A prospective, randomized, double-blind, single center study. Crit Care Med 1999;27:723-732.
27. Chawla, K., Y. Kupfer, I. Goldman, et al. Hydrocortisone reverses refractory septic shock. Crit Care Med 1999;27:A33.
28. ACCP SCCM Consensus Conference Committee. American College of Chest Physicians/ Society of Critical Care Medicine Consensus Conference: Definitions for sepsis and organ failure and guidelines for the use of innovative therapies in sepsis. Critical Care Medicine 1992;20:864-874.
29. Abraham, E., R. Wunderink, H. Silverman, et al. Efficacy and safety of monoclonal antibody to human tumor necrosis factor-alpha in patients with sepsis syndrome. A randomized, controlled, double-blind multi-center clinical trial. TNF-alpha MAb Sepsis Study Group. JAMA 1995;273:934-941.
30. Cohen, J., and J. Carlet. Intersept: An international, multicenter, placebo controlled trial of monoclonal antibody to human tumor necrosis factor-alpha in patients with sepsis. Crit Care Med 1996;24:1431-1440.
31. Abraham, E., A. Anzueto, G. Guterrez, et al. Double-blind randomized controlled trial of monoclonal antibody to human tumor necrosis factor in human septic shock. Lancet 1998;351:929-933.
32. Clark, M., L. Plank, A. Connolly, et al. Effect of a chimeric antibody to tumor necrosis factor alpha on cytokine and physiologic responses in patients with severe sepsis. A randomized clinical trial. Crit Care Med 1998;26:1650-1659.
33. Rheinhart, K., C. Wiegland-Lohnart, F. Grimmanger, et al. Assessment of the safety and efficacy of the monoclonal antitumor necrosis factor antibody-fragment MAK 19F

in patients with sepsis and septic shock: a multicenter, randomized placebo-controlled study. Crit Care Med 1996;24:733-742.

34. Kay, C. A. Can better measures of cytokine responses be obtained to guide cytokine inhibition? Pressentation and handout Washington DC, Cambridge Health Institutes February 20-1, 1996.
35. Dhainaut, J., J. Vincent, C. Richard, et al. CD571, a humanized antibody to tumor necrosis factor-alpha: safety, pharmacodynamics, immune responses and influence of the antibody on cytokine concentrations in patients with septic shock. Crit Care Med 1995;21:1461-1469.
36. Fisher, C., S. Opal, J. Dhainaut, et al. The CB006 Sepsis Syndrome Study Group. Crit Care Med 1993;21:318-327.
37. Abraham, E., M. Glauser, T. Butler, et al. P55 tumor nerosis factor receptor fusion protein in the treatment of patients with septic shock. JAMA 1997;277:1531-1538.
38. Abraham, E. Immunomodulatory therapy in sepsis: failure in clinical trials or critical thinking. International Conference, American Thoracic Society, Chicago, Illinois Tuesday April 28, 1998.
39. Fisher, C., J. Agosti, S. Opal, et al. Treatment of septic shock with the tumor necrosis factor receptor Fc fusion protein. N Engl J Med 1997;334:1697-1702.
40. Fisher, C., G. Slotman, S. Opal, et al. Initial evaluation of human recombinant interleukin-1 receptor antagonist in the treatment of sepsis syndrome: a randomized, open label, placebo controlled clinical trial. Crit Care Med 1994;22:12-21.
41. Opal, S., C. Fisher, F. Dhainaut, et al. Confirmatory interleuken-1 receptor antagonist in severe sepsis: a phase III, randomized double-blind, placebo controlled,multi-center trial. Crit Care Med 1997;25:1115-1124.
42. Fisher, C., J. Dhainaut, and S. Opal. Recombinant human interleukin-1 receptor antagonist in the treatment of patients with the sepsis syndrome. JAMA 1994;271:1836-1848.
43. Dhainaut, J., A. Tenaillon, Y. deTulzo, et al. Platelet-activating factor receptor antagonist BN 52021 in the treatment of severe sepsis: A randomized, placebo controlled, multi-center clinical trial. Crit Care Med 1994;22:1720-1728.
44. Dhainaut, J., A. Tenaillon, M. Hemmer, et al. The confirmatory platelet-activating factor receptor antagonist trial in patients with severe gram negative bacterial sepsis: a multi-center, randomized, placebo controlled, multicenter trial. Crit Care Med 1998;26:1963-1971.
45. Rodell, T., and C. Foster. Sepsis data show negative trend in second phase II sepsis trial. Press Release. Cortec, Inc, 7000 North Broadway, Denver CO 80821 July 18, 1995.
46. Fein, A., G. Bernard, G. Criner, et al. Treatment of severe systemic inflammatory response syndrome and sepsis with a novel bradykinin antagonist, deltibant (CP-O127): results of a randomized, double-blind, placebo controlled trial. JAMA 1997;277:482-7.
47. Jacobs, E., M. Soulsby, R. Bone, et al. Ibuprofen in canine endotoxin shock. J Clin Invest 1982;70:536-71.
48. Wright, P. E., and G. R. Bernard. Mechanisms of late hemodynamic and airway dynamic responses to endotoxin in awake sheep. Am Rev Resp Dis 1989;140:672-678.
49. Bernard, G., A. Wheeler, J. Russel, et al. The effects of ibuprofen on the physiology and survival of patients with sepsis. The ibuprofen in sepsis study group. N Engl J Med 1997;336:912-8.

50. Haupt, M., M. Jastremski, T. Clemmer, et al. Effect of ibuprofen in patients with severe sepsis; a randomized, double-blind multi-center trial. Crit Care Med 1991;19:1339-1347.
51. Sevransky, J. E., and C. Natanson. An analysis of clinical trials of mediator-specific anti-inflammatory agents. Sepsis 1999;3:11-19.
52. Natanson, C., C. Esposito, and S. M. Banks. The siren's song of confirmatory sepsis trials; selection bias and sampling error. Crit Care Med 1998;26:1927-1931.
53. Natanson, C., P. W. Eichenholz, and R. L. Danner. Endotoxin and tumor necrosis factor challenges in dogs simulate the cardiovascular profile of human septic shock. J Exp Med 1989;169:823-832.
54. Suffredini, A. F., R. E. Fromm, M. M. Parker, et al. The cardiovascular response of normal humans to the administration of endotoxin. N Engl J Med 1989;321:280-287.
55. Natanson, H. W., Suffredini AF, Eichacker PQ, and Danner RL. Selected Treatment Strategies for Septic Shock Based on Proposed Mechanisms of Pathogenesis. Ann Int Med 1994;120:771-783.
56. Ziegler, E. J., J. A. McCutchan, and J. Fierer. Treatment of gram-negative bacteremia and shock with human antiserum to a mutant Esherichia coli. N Engl J Med 1982;307:1225-1230.
57. Ziegler, E. J., C. J. Fisher, and C. L. Sprung. Treatment of gram-negative bacteremia and septic shock with HA-1A human monoclonal antibody against endotoxin. New Engl J Med 1991;324:429-426.
58. The J5 Study Group. Treatment of severe infectious purpura in children with human plasma from donors immunized with Esherichia coli J5: a prospective double-blind study. J Infect Dis 1992;165:695-701.
59. Calandra, T., M. P. Glauser, J. Schellekens, et al. Treatment of gram-negative septic shock with human IgG antibody to Escherichia coli J5; a prospective, double-blind, randomized trial. J Infect Dis 1988;158:312-319.
60. Greenman, R. L., R. M. H. Scein, and M. A. Martin. A controlled clinical trial of E5 murine monoclonal IgM antibody to endotoxin in the treatment of gram-negative sepsis. JAMA 1991;266:1097-1102.
61. Bone, R. C., R. A. Balk, and A. M. Fein. A second large controlled clinical study of E5, a monoclonal antibody to endotoxin: results of a prospective, multicenter, randomized, controlled trial. Crit Care Med 1995;23:994-1006.
62. McClosky, R. V., R. C. Straube, C. Sanders, et al. Treatment of septic shock with human monoclonal antibody HA-1A. Ann Int Med 121: 1-5, 1994.
63. McCutchan, J. A., J. L. Wolf, E. L. Ziegler, et al. Ineffectiveness of single-dose human antiserum to core glycolipid (Esherichia coli J5) for prophylaxis of bacteremic, gram-negative infection in patients with prolonged neutropenia. J Suisse de Medecine 1983;113(s):40-55.
64. The Intravenous Immunoglobulin Collaborative Study Group. Prophylactic intravenous administration of standard immune globulin compared with core-lipopolysaccaride immune globulin in patients at high risk of post-surgical infection. N Engl J Med 1992;327:234-40.
65. Baumgartner, J. D., D. Heumann, J. Gerain, et al. Association between protective efficacy of anti-lipopolysaccharide (LPS) antibodies and suppression of LPS-induced tumor necrosis factor alpha and interleukin 6. Comparison of O side chain-specific antibodies with core LPS antibodies. J Exp Med 1990;171:889-896.
66. Baumgartner, J. D. Immunotherapy with antibodies to core lipopolysaccharide: a critical appraisal. Infect Dis Clinics NA 1991;5:915-917.

67. Aiki, H., M. Kodama, T. Tani, et al. Treatment of sepsis by extracorporeal elimination of endotoxin using polymyxin B-immobilized fiber. Am J Surgery 1994;167:412-4171994.
68. Bernard GR, Reines HD, Haluska DV. Prostacyclin and thromboxone A2 formatica is increased in human sepsis syndrome: effects of cyclooxygenase inhibition. Am Rev Respir Dis 1991;144:1095-1101.
69. Lucas CE, Ledgerwood AN. The cardiopulmonary response to massive doses of steroids in patients with septic shock. Arch Surg 1984;119:537-541.

Chapter 10

PERSPECTIVES IN ANTI-INFLAMMATORY THERAPIES IN SEPSIS

Jean-François Dhainaut, M.D., Ph.D., Nathalie Marin, Ph.D., Alain Cariou, M.D.
Medical Intensive Care Unit, Cochin Port-Royal University Hospital

Introduction

Sepsis represents a systemic reaction to a microbial infection. The reaction is triggered by bacterial toxins or by components of microbial cell wall fragments. Innate immunity with its germ-line encoded receptors for the recognition of microbial pathogens, represents a phylogenetically ancient defense against micro-organisms. Acquired immunity allows the development of memory of previously encountered pathogens, and results from the generation of a large repertoire of antigen-recognizing receptors.

Severe sepsis occurs when over stimulation of the innate immune response results in excessive release of inflammatory mediators and activation of multiple complex proteolytic cascades. Such a defensive response, although eliminating bacterial toxins and infection, may itself result in tissue injury and death (1). In the USA, more than half a million patients develop severe sepsis each year, and approximately 40% of these patients die (2-3). Moreover, the management of sepsis has other significant economic consequences by increasing length of ICU stay and resource use. As a result of this, a great deal of attention has been paid to defining management strategies that could improve outcome with sepsis.

Conventional treatment for sepsis consists of prompt resuscitation and physiologic support, eradication of the source of infection, and appropriate antimicrobial therapy (3). Based on our growing understanding regarding the important role an excessive host defensive response has in the organ injury and mortality of sepsis, recent research has also been directed at the application of immunomodulatory therapies (3). However, despite initially encouraging results in laboratory animals and in several phase II clinical trials, immunomodulatory agents have invariably not been shown to significantly improve survival in large clinical trials. This disappointing experience with immmunomodulatory therapies in sepsis is in striking contrast to our successful experience with similar agents directed against proinflammatory cytokines (e.g. TNF, IL-1) in diseases such as rheumatoid arthritis and Crohn's disease (1).

The failure of immunomodulatory therapies to improve outcome in sepsis raises several important questions about drug development and design of clinical trials in this area. A review of the major clinical trials of immunomodulatory therapies in sepsis provides a perspective on the possible causes for these failures. Such a perspective may help in designing future sepsis trials, particularly with respect to the selection of patients who would theoretically benefit the most from immunomodulatory therapies (2). The purpose of this chapter is to review the lessons learned from large clinical trials in sepsis over the last ten years, and to evaluate current and future therapies aimed at modulating innate immunity in the early and late phases of sepsis.

LESSONS LEARNED IN THE LAST 10 YEARS

Critical analysis of clinical trials

In order to identify new therapeutic targets for the treatment of sepsis, over the past decade more than 17,000 patients were enrolled in at least 35 phase II-III clinical trials testing the effects of immunomodulatory therapies. These agents included high dose corticosteroids, endotoxin directed antibodies, and agents designed to selectively inhibit specific host mediators.

High Dose Corticosteroids: Based on their successful application as pretreatment in animals with endotoxemia or bacteremia, early clinical trials studied the effect of large doses of corticosteroids in patients with septic shock. However, large double blind studies showed no benefit with corticosteroids even when they were administered early in the course of septic shock (4). Recent studies have reported improved survival using much lower doses of corticosteroids in patients with prolonged septic shock or with unresolved sepsis-induced organ system dysfunction (4). This topic is reviewed elsewhere in this volume.

Antiendotoxin Antibodies: Specific anti-endotoxin therapies, such as hyperimmune polyclonal human immunoglobulin G raised against heat killed E.coli J5, and murine (E5) and humanized (HA1A) monoclonal antibodies directed against the lipid A moiety of endotoxin, have been investigated in patients with severe gram-negative infection (5). Although initial clinical results were encouraging, larger trials failed to show benefit with these antibodies, possibly due to their inability to effectively block the effects of endotoxin. More specific anti-endotoxin agents, such as a bactericidal permeability increasing protein (BPI), are now under investigation (6).

Table 1. Clinical trials of non-glucocorticoid mediator-specific anti-inflammatory agents.*

Agents (company)	Phase	Patient population	Control N (%mortality)	Treated N (%mortality)
Anti-TNF MAb				
CB006 (Celltech)	II	Severe sepsis	19 (32%)	61 (44%)
CDP571 (Celltech)	II	Septic shock	10 (60%)	32 (63%)
NORACEPT I (Bayeer)	III	Severe sepsis	326 (33%)	645 (30%)
INTERCEPT (Bayer)	III	Severe sepsis	167 (40%)	386 (37%)
NORACEPT II (Bayer)	III	Septic shock	930 (43%)	948 (40%)
cA2 (Centocor)	II	Severe sepsis	28 (39%)	28 (36%)
MAK 195F (Knoll)	II	Severe sepsis	29 (41%)	93 (47%)
MAK 195F (Knoll)	II	Severe sepsis	12 (50%)	27 (26%)
MAK 195F (Knoll)	III	Sepsis (high IL-6 level)	221 (57%)	225 (54%)
sTNFr				
P75 (Immunex)	II	Septic shock	33 (30%)	108 (45%)
P55 (Roche)	II	Severe sepsis	140 (39%)	358 (38%)
P55 (Roche)	III	Septic shock	680 (28%)	682 (27%)
IL-1ra				
Antril (Synergen)	II	Severe sepsis	25 (44%)	74 (24%)
Antril (Synergen)	III	Severe sepsis	302 (34%)	591 (30%)
Antril (Synergen)	III	Severe sepsis	346 (36%)	350 (33%)
PAFra				
BN 52021 (Ipsen)	III	Severe sepsis	130 (51%)	132 (42%)
BN 52021 (Ipsen)	III	Severe sepsis	308 (49%)	300 (47%)
BB-882 (British Biotech)	II	Severe sepsis	69 (45%)	83 (53%)
Anti-prostaglandin				
Ibuprofen (Upjohn)	II	Severe sepsis	13 (31%)	16 (56%)
Ibuprofen (Upjohn)	II	Severe sepsis	14 (43%)	16 (19%)
Ibuprofen (Upjohn)	III	Severe sepsis	231 (40%)	224 (37%)
Anti-bradykinin				
CPO127 (Cortech)	II	Sepsis	84 (29%)	167 (37%)
CPO127 (Cortech)	II	Sepsis	126 (36%)	378 (39%)

- See references 2 and 15 for the references of all clinical trials of non-glucocorticoid mediator-specific anti-inflammatory agents.

Mediator-Specific Immunomodulatory Agents, Anti-TNF Therapies: Among non-glucorticoid mediator-specific anti-inflammatory agents (Table 1), anti-TNF therapies were the first strategy used, and included anti-TNF monoclonal antibodies (MAb) and soluble TNF receptors. TNF is the proinflammatory mediator most identified with the pathophysiology of sepsis. TNF administration reproduces many of the manifestations of sepsis in animal models. Also, treatment with MAb against TNF improves survival rates in many sepsis models. There have been nine published clinical trials with anti-TNF MAbs of which five were double-blinded. None of these single trials showed a significant reduction in mortality in rats. When results from these studies were pooled, a small non-significant trend towards reduced mortality could be noted : 42% v.s. 39%, p = 0.14 (2). The preliminary results of a recent phase III study using an anti-TNF MAb do appear encouraging however (E. Panacek, personal communication, see below). Soluble TNF receptors (sTNFr) which are naturally shed from cells into the circulation and can be produced by biologic engineering techniques, were used as a second anti-TNF approach. Three double-blinded studies showed no treatment benefit, and a large-molecular weight sTNFr even increased mortality in a small trial (2).

IL-1 Receptor Antagonist (IL-1ra): The cytokine IL-1 also reproduces many of the clinical manifestations of sepsis. These effects can be blocked by IL-1ra, a natural IL-1 receptor antagonist produced by various types of cells, including macrophages. Three trials (two double-blinded) performed in patients with severe sepsis showed no survival difference between the treatment and placebo arms. When the studies were analyzed together, there was a small trend towards decreased mortality in IL-1ra-treated patients: 36 vs. 31%, p = 0.10 (2).

PAF Receptor Antagonist (PAFra): Platelet aggregating factor (PAF) is a phospholipid that has been implicated in the release of cytokines during ARDS and sepsis. Two double-blinded studies performed with a PAF receptor antagonist (BN 52021) showed no significant improvement in survival. However, among mediator-specific antiinflammatory agents, the trend towards a beneficial effect with this treatment has been the largest one thus far observed: 50 vs. 45% mortality rate (2). Recently, a phase II trial using another compound (BB-882) again showed no significant improvement in survival for patients with severe sepsis. Another PAF antagonist, PAF-acetyl hydrolase, has shown promising early results in a phase II sepsis trial (J. Pribble, personal communication).

Non-steroidal Anti-inflammatory Agents: Ibuprofen, an anti-prostaglandin agent, was tested in three double-blinded trials. Benefit with ibuprofen could not be demonstrated in any of these trials. The mortality rate was not significantly different between the two treatment arms, even when data from the 3 studies were pooled: 40 vs. 37%, p = 0.14 (2).

Bradykinin Antagonists: Bradykinin is a bioactive peptide that has been implicated in the release of cytokines and in vascular alterations in sepsis. Two double-blinded studies showed no improvement in mortality rate with a bradykinin antagonist (2).

Overall therefore, none of these trials individually showed a significant beneficial effect with mediator-specific immunomodulatory agents. However, when data from these six agents were pooled, a relatively modest (<10%) but significant beneficial treatment effect on survival rate was observed (39 vs 36%, p = 0.023). If one can assume that these six agents represent a single uniform class of agent, this result suggests that there may be some validity in the use of antiinflammatory agents for sepsis. This does not however allow us to make inferences or draw any conclusions about an individual trial (2). It has been calculated by Natanson et al. that in order to demonstrate a survival benefit for any of these anti-inflammatory agents, a sepsis trial would require a very large enrollment (i.e. 6,000 to 7,000 patients). Consequently, understanding why these trials have failed in sepsis may help us better select patient populations for this therapeutic approach as well as better direct our research for more effective agents.

WHY HAVE SEPSIS TRIALS FAILED?

Sepsis trials may have failed for several reasons. The drugs tested may have been ineffective. The targets chosen may have been the wrong ones. Clinical trial design may have been inappropriate. The failure of these trials raises other questions however related to issues such as the animal models used for preclinical testing and our ability to clearly characterize the critical elements defining the septic patient likely to respond to a particular type of treatment.

Some of the agents tested may have had insufficient activity clinically. This may have been because they either lacked absolute biological activity or because they were inactivated in vivo by other mediators. Alternatively, despite the activity of agents against specific intermediary host mediators like cytokines (e.g. TNF or IL-1), independent activation of other injurious host systems (e.g. coagulation or complement cascades) during sepsis may have bypassed the potentially beneficial effects of some agents. It is also possible that death in some septic patients, such as those with severe underlying disease like heart failure, may have been related to factors independent of the inflammatory response itself. In such patients, inhibiting inflammatory mediators may have done little to determine clinical outcome. It is also possibility that genetic variability in the level of expression of host inflammatory mediators like TNF may have caused agents to be beneficial in some patients, but harmful in others (7).

The disparity between the beneficial effects of antiinflammatory agents in preclinical models and our disappointing clinical experience raises important questions about the relevance of these models. It is likely that differences between the biochemical and immunologic responses of patients with a clinical diagnosis of sepsis and animals with known bacterial infections or endotoxemia may explain the disparity in results comparing experimental and clinical studies. In animal models, the cascade of events starting from the initial stimulus until death follows a predictable and usually rapid time course. The resulting cytokine production in such models occurs in a recognized pattern and can be controlled (8). Therefore, affecting outcome in animal models by blocking one or another cytokine in an activated cascade is relatively easy. The sequence of events leading to septic shock and sepsis-related organ injury in humans appears much more complex. Critical care physicians have recognized for a long time that many septic patients have a long and complicated course of disease, little resembling that of animal models. For example, a patient admitted with fecal peritonitis who seems to initially progress towards recovery may later relapse as a consequence of secondary complications (e.g. ventilator-associated pneumonia or intra-abdominal abscess formation). There are two other caveats that preclude generalization from animal studies. Blocking the actions of pro-inflammatory cytokines is usually successful when given before the challenge. Cytokine blockade is particularly effective when the toxic challenge is hyperacute, as exemplified by intravenous administration of a bolus containing billions of *E.coli* or a large amount of endotoxin. Indeed, even in animal models, if the challenge is subacute, as with peritonitis (e.g. cecal ligation and puncture) or pneumonitis, cytokine blockade has been mostly unsuccessful or harmful (1,8,9). In humans, sites and types of bacterial infection are very diverse. Also, patients have a large variety of underlying diseases. Finally, patients routinely receive other therapies which may themselves lead to adverse reactions (9) such as: antibiotics (endotoxin release), narcotic agents (increased risk of nosocomial infections), dopamine (antagonism of prolactin secretion), beta-adrenergic agonists (anti-inflammatory agents), allogeneic red blood cell transfusions (immunosuppression), etc.

Our poor experience with antiinflammatory agents in sepsis is in striking contrast to the beneficial effects noted with these agents (e.g. anti-TNF MAbs) in several well defined diseases (e.g. Crohn's disease and rheumatoid arthritis) clearly characterized by inflammatory tissue injury. This difference highlights the probable heterogeneous nature of the pathogenetic mechanisms present in a large population of patients identified as being septic. Thus, whereas rheumatoid arthritis and Crohn's disease are well described entities with specific immunologic, radiologic, and pathophysiologic diagnostic criteria, the defining features of sepsis are based mainly on organ system dysfunction developing in the appropriate clinical setting (1). Overly broad definitions for sepsis may have negated the demonstration of any beneficial effect with antiinflammatory agents that would have only been possible in a more tightly defined patient population.

The inclusion criteria used for many sepsis trials were based on the consensus definition of sepsis developed by the ACCP/SCCM. Although these criteria have been conceptually useful, they are non-specific. Poor understanding of the nonspecific nature of these criteria may have lead some investigators to enroll nonseptic patients inappropriately in sepsis trials. The ACCP/SCCM criteria may also be too restrictive, excluding some severely infected patients unable to demonstrate necessary entry criteria such as fever. Thus, these criteria may not only be nonspecific but also insensitive for the identification of patients with septic shock (1).

Both the presence or absence and type of actual infection in patients enrolled in clinical sepsis trials may have also influenced the effects of antiinflammatory agents. Entry criteria for these trials were designed primarily to include patients with clinical evidence of infection associated with the recent development of infection related organ dysfunction. In addition though, because of the perceived need to enroll patients early in their clinical course, positive microbiological cultures were not required in many trials. However, in a number of recent studies, only a minority (i.e. 30%) of patients enrolled ultimatley were found to have positive blood cultures (1). This number is in fact much lower than the expected incidence of positive blood cultures (i.e. 50 – 60%) for such a patient population as determined in observational studies. The lack of a requirement to recruit patients with documented infection may have therefore adversely affected outcome in trials examining the potential benefit of immunomodulatory agents in sepsis. This possibility is supported by the improved efficacy of antiinflammatory therapies (e.g. anti-TNF MAb), noted when blinded data safety monitoring committees eliminated patients in studies without clear evidence of infection (12). The definition of sepsis used in most clinical trials also did not include the length of time that the infective process had been present, nor its anatomic site. As emphasized above, such a classification may be particularly important since animal studies have shown different patterns of response to anti-cytokine therapies for more slowly developing intra-abdominal or intra-pulmonary infections compared to more rapidly developing primary intravascular bacteremia (1,8,9). Furthermore, no microbiological classifications were used prospectively in clinical trials of immunomodulatory agents even though responses to anti-inflammatory therapies may not only be more pronounced in the setting of documented infection but may also differ comparing gram-positive and gram-negative infections (10).

Even though endotoxin, TNF, IL-1, and PAF were identified as pivotal mediators in the pathophysiology of sepsis and targeted in recent clinical trials, their actual presence in excessive levels was not required for entry into study. Rather, clinical criteria such as the presence of one or more organ failures with or without the presence shock were used. Although elevation of the mediator of interest was postulated to accompany organ system dysfunction in septic patients, data gathered from IL-1ra and anti-TNF clinical outcome in trials examining trials suggested that such a correlation was present in only a minority of cases. For example, in the NORASEPT II study (anti-TNF MAb tested in patients with septic shock), only 40% of patients had detectable circulating TNF levels at the time of enrollment (1). Thus the lack of a requirement to recruit patients with elevated plasma levels of the mediator the investigational agent was directed against may have also adversely affected the potential benefit of immunomodulatory agents in these sepsis trials. In support of this, in the NORASEPT II trial, patients with detectable circulating TNF levels at time of enrollment receiving the MAb had an 18% reduction in mortality compared to placebo (1). By contrast, no effect of the anti-TNF treatment was observed in patients without elevated circulating TNF concentrations. As stated above, the preliminary results of a new phase III study with an anti-TNF MAb are encouraging. In this phase III trial, bedside measurements of IL-6 may have been useful in the selection of patients responsive to therapy (E. Panacek, personal communication). Interestingly however, a similar approach (bedside IL-6 as criteria for enrollment) failed in a phase III trial testing another anti-TNF MAb (MAK 195, Knoll).

Is mortality a realistic endpoint in sepsis trials ? The question of outcome is a controversial one. At present, 28-day all-cause mortality has been taken as the gold standard for efficacy: a drug is considered valuable only if the 28-day mortality is significantly reduced. Cohen et al (8) raised the following question: "Are the academic community and the regulatory authorities in danger of making a type II error, overlooking the possibility of a beneficial effect by making such stringent demands?" We are dealing with a complex disease, and we should not necessarily expect simple answers. Many experts believe that morbidity end points such as organ failure-free days, ventilator-free days, need for dialysis, etc. should replace mortality in future clinical trials. In addition, increasing survival time without improving overall survival rates may only translate into additional time in the intensive care unit without any improvement in quality of life but an increase in the utilization of critical care resources.

Several other explanations as to why a given study drug failed have been published in recent reviews. It is possible that variations in the timing (e.g. to early or late) or method (e.g. appropriate dose or duration) of administration of antiinflammatory agents may have altered their effects in clinical trials (11). It is also possible that study populations were overly heterogeneous with respect to the presence or absence of concurrent therapies including adequacy of surgical source control, antimicrobials, and concomitant intensive care unit supportive care. Specific evidence for such problems was found when a Clinical Evaluation Committee reviewed patient management in sepsis trials in detail (12).

NEW RECOMMENDATIONS FOR FUTURE TRIALS

There is no doubt that we have learned much from our experience with clinical trials in sepsis. A simple comparison of the design of a sepsis trial with large doses of corticosteroids performed 15 years ago with one of the recent studies with a mediator-specific agent demonstrates this very well. We now are very careful to take into account factors which may have a major impact on outcome such as risk assessment, severity of underlying disease, appropriateness of antimicrobial therapy, adequacy of surgery, etc. However, our experience also provides a basis for additional recommendations for future trials.

The use of ACCP/SCCM criteria (1) to define patient populations who are at risk for infection-initiated organ system dysfunction should be refined or replaced by more specific, understandable, and reproducible definitions. Because of substantial differences in the intracellular signaling cascades initiated by gram-negative and gram-positive infections (10), as well as by the site of infection (1,8,9), it would be reasonable to limit the nature and site of infection in patients enrolled in future trials of immunomodulatory agents (1). For example, an immunomodulatory therapy might initially be investigated only in those patients with meningococcemia or pneumococcal pneumonia. Positive results associated with anti-TNF therapy for the prevention of the Jarisch-Herxheimer reaction (1) or with endotoxin blockade for meningococcemia (6), suggest that specific groups of infected patients may be much more sensitive to the beneficial effects of some immunomodulatory agents.

Rapid diagnostic tests in microbiology, such as the polymerase chain reaction (PCR), may accelerate and increase the sensitivity of bacterial testing. Such testing might better ensure the early and accurate enrollment of patients with documented infection in trials.

Classification of infected patients based on demonstrable abnormalities in immunologic, inflammatory or biochemical pathways may allow inclusion of a more homogeneous population at earlier points of their clinical course, before organ dysfunction becomes irreversible. These tests could focus on the specific mediator the investigational agent was designed to inhibit or replace. Plasma endotoxin levels could be measured in a study aimed at blocking endotoxin. Plasma TNF or IL-6 levels could be determined in a trial of an anti-TNF MAb. Plasma AT-III or activated protein C concentrations could be measured if these factors were to be therapeutically replaced (13). The hypothalamic-adrenal axis could be dynamically evaluated (14) in a corticosteroid trial. Improved techniques to monitor immunologic markers of inflammatory and host defense responses will be key in assessing the effects of future therapies on central mechanisms contributing to organ dysfunction in sepsis (15).

With regards to outcome, the use of 14 and 28 day survival as end points should be rexamined. Information on long-term outcome (e.g. 3 months or more) with respect to quality of life and resource utilization and cost will be crucial in future sepsis trials.

Undoubtedly "clinical evaluation committees" markedly improve the quality of trials (12). These committees analyze the validity of entry and exclusion criteria, the severity of underlying disorders, the microbiological data, the adequacy of antimicrobial therapy and surgery, as well as the cause of death. Institution of such committees should be standard in trials.

Finally, future clinical trials will likely benefit from implementation of protocols that ensure uniform administration of concurrent therapies such antimicrobial agents and hemodynamic and ventilatory support. Ensuring such uniformity should be standard whenever possible.

FUTURE DIRECTIONS IN MODULATING INNATE IMMUNITY

Given the relatively modest treatment effect mediator-specific anti-inflammatory agents have demonstrated, we must continue our search for more effective agents. As stated above, these disappointing results do not negate the validity of therapeutically modulating the inflammatory response to infection. Indeed, microbial cell wall components stimulate inflammation and toxic reactions, not only indirectly through the release of cytokines, but also directly by stimulating pathways such as those involving nitric oxide, coagulation/fibrinolysis, and complement. While blocking cytokine action can modulate the former processes, such blockade does not interrupt cascades that have been activated directly. In this regard, we suggest that therapies designed to inhibit the direct effects of microbial toxins (e.g. antagonists of the Toll-like receptors) as well as direct modulation of other major pathways (e.g. nitric oxide, coagulation and complement) be tested. We believe it will be important to test therapies separately that are designed to either block the early effects of microbial products on host receptors (Toll-like receptors) or the later effects of major host pathways (e.g. nitric oxide, coagulation, and complement). In addition, other host mediators like macrophage migration inhibitory factor (MIF) and high mobility group-1 (HMG-1) protein have recently been identified which appear to be important in the pathogenesis of tissue injury and death occurring late in the inflammatory response. The plasma levels of these mediators peak more slowly after the onset of sepsis that the "classical" pro-inflammatory cytokines. They therefore represent other attractive targets for future therapeutic intervention.

AT THE EARLY PHASE OF SEPSIS

Toll-like receptors

The molecular and cellular processes involved in triggering an inflammatory reaction have been recently well defined. Gram-negative bacterial endotoxin binds to a specific plasma acute phase protein (lipopolysaccharide-binding protein, LBP), and this complex binds the macrophage membrane CD14 receptor. Endotoxin is then presented to another receptor, recently identified as Toll-like receptor (TLR) 4, which promotes transmembrane signaling (16). Gram-positive organisms can trigger sepsis by superantigens and, more frequently, by cell wall components that bind to another member of the TLR family, TLR2. TLRs and CD14 represent attractive therapeutic targets, since their blockade may blunt cytokine release in response to both gram-negative and gram-positive bacteria.

Filtration of mediators

Blood purification via mechanical filtration has also been proposed as a therapy in sepsis. It has been hypothesized that an excessive inflammatory response could be neutralized with hemofiltration, especially using high flow and large-pore hemofilters. However, the evidence for the clinically effective elimination of inflammatory mediators, as well as evidence for a beneficial effect of hemofiltration on outcome remains poor (17). In contrast, plasma filtration coupled with adsorption techniques may be more efficient for the removal of endotoxin and cytokines. The clinical experience with this method is limited thus far however (18).

Inhibitors of inducible nitric oxide synthase (iNOS)

Nitric oxide (NO), a free radical gas produced by numerous cell types, is implicated in a wide range of disease processes, exerting both detrimental and beneficial effects at the cellular and vascular levels. NO is synthesized intracellularly by the oxidation of L-arginine as catalyzed by nitric oxide synthases (NOS). These enzymes exist in a constitutive and calcium dependent (cNOS) form and in an inducible and calcium independent (iNOS) one. iNOS expression can be induced by specific proinflammatory agents in many types of cells. Once produced, NO can react with the superoxide anion to form peroxynitrite (ONOO•), a powerful oxidant with toxic effects on many molecules including nucleic acids, lipids and proteins. In different animal models, sepsis has been shown to increase the constitutive release of NO by the endothelium and the activity of the iNOS enzyme (19). In such conditions, limiting the indirect effects of NO may be a viable therapeutic option to reduce tissue injury and improve survival. At the same time, maintenance or enhancement of the direct effects of NO may be suitable to reduce antioxidant-mediated organ damage, improve tissue perfusion and reduce leukocyte adhesion and platelet aggregation.

The preclinical data for this approach was more equivocal than for other strategies since blocking NO increased mortality in some animal models. Furthermore, despite encouraging results in a small phase II study with a nonspecific competitive inhibitor of NOS (L-N-monomethyl arginine, L-NMMA), a larger phase III trial had to be stopped prematurely due to increased mortality in the treatment group (15, 20).

A viable strategy to modulate the effects of NO should protect its positive effects while eradicating its negative ones. Selective iNOS inhibitors may achieve this better than nonselective agents, but these compounds have not undergone clinical testing yet. It may be that different agents are needed at different times during the septic process, or that a combination of NO inhibitors with NO donors may be needed (20). Other approaches include therapies aimed at limiting peroxynitrite generation (e.g. scavengers). Such agents should be efficient in removing excess NO, superoxide anion and peroxynitrite. Although specific peroxynitrite scavengers are still in relatively early stages of development, it is noteworthy that the recently developed compound mercaptoethylguanidine, which combines properties of selective iNOS inhibition and peroxynitrite scavenging, has been shown to provide significant benefits in experimental models of inflammation and shock (21).

Oxygen free radical scavengers

Excessive production of oxygen free radicals are implicated in endothelial cell damage and multiple organ failure during septic shock. Nacetylcysteine is one of the most important endogenous antioxidants. It has been used with promising results in patients with septic shock (15). No large clinical trials have been performed thus far however.

Coagulation/fibrinolysis pathway

During sepsis, bacterial components and pro-inflammatory cytokines induce the expression of tissue factor (TF) on monocytes and endothelial cells. This promotes the activation of the extrinsic coagulation pathway and the consumption of coagulation factors and their endogenous inhibitors, leading to disseminated intravascular coagulation (DIC). Thrombosis of the microvasculature associated with DIC is currently believed to play a significant role in organ dysfunction related to sepsis. Regulatory mechanisms that prevent coagulation from being generalized under normal conditions involve tissue factor pathway inhibitor (TFPI), antithrombin III (AT III), and protein C. Each of these inhibitory mechanisms is presently being investigated as a therapeutic intervention to improve outcome from severe sepsis.

TFPI is an endogenous antagonist of the extrinsic pathway of coagulation that inhibits factor Xa directly and the factor VIIa/TF catalytic complex. Administration of TFPI improved survival and organ function when given to rabbits with septic peritonitis and to baboons infused with E.coli. It was effective even when given several hours after the insult and in doses lacking significant anticoagulant effect. TFPI was found to also exhibit anti-inflammatory activities as reflected by decreases of IL-6 and IL-8 plasma levels in the treated animals. It is well tolerated in human volunteers, although high doses increased thromboplastin time. In contrast to a high dose pilot study, a new phase II study using low doses was not associated with bleeding complications, and showed a trend toward improvement of survival (22). Consequently, a phase III trial using low doses is underway.

AT III is a major inhibitor of the coagulation system which blocks activated proteases, including factors IXa, Xa and thrombin. Plasma levels of AT III decrease in animals and humans with sepsis, and inversely correlate with survival. AT III infusion to supraphysiologic concentrations may offer protection against DIC and related morbidity. Importantly, this strategy provided a survival advantage in multiple animal species with sepsis, but high doses were required to compensate for the increased AT III consumption associated with this syndrome. Despite several positive phase II trials (23), a large phase III trial recently showed no improvement of mortality in patients with severe sepsis.

Protein C is a vitamin K-dependent protein, which is activated by the thrombin-thrombomodulin complex at the surface of endothelial cells. The activated form of protein C (APC) functions as an anticoagulant with its cofactor, protein S, by inactivating factors Va and VIIIa, thereby blocking the generation of thrombin. Recombinant human APC (rhAPC) and plasma-derived APC have been shown to significantly improve organ failure and survival in animal models of septic shock. Depressed protein C levels have been associated with a sustained procoagulant state during sepsis, sepsis-induced acute lung injury, trauma, and meningococcemia. Protein C levels inversely correlated with survival, with levels being a strong predictor of outcome in human sepsis. A phase II trial testing high doses of APC provided promising results (24). Preliminary results of a large phase III trial performed in patients with severe sepsis indicate a statistically significant improvement in mortality rate (Eli Lilly, press release, July 2000). Although we are waiting for detailed results of this study, it is the first time that such a strategy has been able to reduce mortality in patients with severe sepsis.

Complement blockade

It is generally accepted that the complement system provides essential protection against bacteria through generation of the opsonic factor, C3b, which promotes phagocytosis and intracellular killing of bacteria. The low-molecular-weight anaphylatoxin C5a is a potent agonist for neutrophils and endothelial cells, and increases vasodilation and vascular permeability. In a peritonitis model in rats, anti-C5a treament was able to reduce levels of bacteremia, the H_2O_2 response of blood neutrophils, and mortality rate (25).

AT THE LATE PHASE OF SEPSIS

Low doses of glucocorticoids

Small randomized studies provided the theoretical basis for the use of low-doses of glucocorticoids during the late phase of sepsis (4). We are now waiting for the results of larger ongoing trials as discussed elsewhere in this volume.

Macrophage Migration Inhibitory Factor (MIF)

MIF, a pleiotropic cytokine released by macrophages, T cells and the pituitary gland has emerged as a pivotal cytokine in the innate immune system and the control of the inflammatory response. It is capable of overriding the "anti-inflammatory" effects of glucocorticoids. Once released, MIF induces the expression of proinflammatory mediators by macrophages and activated T cells, thereby promoting inflammatory and immune responses. In fact, it has been shown to act as a proinflammatory cytokine, playing a major role in endotoxin shock and peritonitis as well. Neutralization of MIF prevented death in this model, even when the treatment was begun as long as 8 hours after the onset of peritonitis. The progressive appearance of MIF in peritoneal fluid and blood may explain why treatment with antibody against MIF remained efficacious when given post-infection (26). The ability of delayed administration of antibody against MIF to protect mice from death thus fulfills an essential prerequisite for any anti-sepsis agent, as treatment is almost always started after the onset of infection in patients. This topic is discussed in another chapter of this volume.

High Mobility Group-1 (HMG-1)

Recently, data concerning another potential late mediator of lethality was published. High mobility group-1 (HMG-1) protein was found to be released by cultured macrophages more than 8 hours after stimulation with endotoxin, TNF, or IL-1. Delayed administration of antibodies to HMG-1 attenuated endotoxin lethality in mice. Septic patients who succumbed to infection had increased serum HMG-1 levels, suggesting that this protein warrants investigation as a therapeutic target (27).

CONCLUSIONS

Revolutionary changes in molecular genetics and cell biology promise dramatic changes in medical practice over the next several decades. It will be vital to translate recent advances in the basic sciences into diagnostic tools and treatments which might be applicable for the improved care of patients with sepsis. Any such advances however will have to be carefully tested clinically. Both basic scientists and physicians will have to work closely to provide the necessary bridge from bench to bedside. It is very encouraging at this time to note that such cooperation has resulted in the possible successful application of activated protein C, a compound which influences both anticoagulant/fibrinolysis and inflammatory cascades, to reduce mortality in patients with severe sepsis.

REFERENCES

1. Abraham E. Why immunomodulatory therapies have not worked in sepsis? Intensive Care Med 1999;25:556-566.
2. Sevransky JE, Natanson C. An analysis of clinical trials of mediator-specific anti-inflammatory agents. Sepsis 1999;3:11-19.
3. Wheeler AP, Bernard GR. Treating patients with severe sepsis N Engl J Med 1999;340:207-214.
4. Meduri GU. An historical review of glucocortcoid treatment in sepsis. Sepsis 1999;3:21-38.
5. Llewelyn M, Cohen J. Anti-endotoxin antibodies in sepsis: a critical evaluation. Sepsis 1999;3:39-45.
6. Giroir BP, Quint PA, Barton P, Kirsh EA, Kitchen L, Goldstein B, Nelson BJ, Wedel NJ, Carroll SF, Scannon PJ. Preliminary evaluation of recombinant amino-terminal fragment of human bactericidal/permeability-increasing protein in children with severe meningococcal sepsis.Lancet 1997;350:1439-1443.
7. Mira JP, Cariou A, Grall F, Delclaux C, Losser MR, Heshmati F, Cheval C, Monchi M, Reboul JL, Riche F, Leleu G, Arbibe L, Mignon A, Delpech M, Dhainaut JF. Association of TNF2, a TNF-α promoter polymorphism, with septic shock susceptibility and mortality. JAMA 1999;282:561-568.
8. Cohen J, Heumann D, Glauser MP. Do monoclonal antibodies and anticytokines still have a future in infectious disease. Am J Med 1995;99:45S-51S.
9. Chaudry IH. Sepsis: lessons learned in the last century and future directions. Arch Surg 1999;134:922-929.
10. Opal SM, Cohen J. Are there fundamental differences of clinical relevance between gram-positive and gram-negative bacterial sepsis? Crit Care Med 1999;27:1608-1616.
11. Vincent JL. Search for effective immunomodulating strategies against sepsis. Lancet 1999;351:922-923.
12. Sprung C, Finch RG, Thijs LG, Glauser MP. International sepsis trial (INTERSEPT): role and impact of a clinical evaluation committee. Crit Care Med 1996;24:1441-1447.
13. Esmon CT. New potential therapeutic modalities: aPC. Sepsis 1999;3:161-172.
14. Annane D, Seville V, Troche G, Raphael JC, Gajdos P, Bellissant E. A 3-level prognostic classification in septic shock based on cortisol levels and cortisol response to corticotropin. JAMA 2000;283:1038-1045.
15. Cohen J. Adjunctive therapy in sepsis; a critical analysis of the clinical programme. Br Med Bull 1999;55:212-225.
16. Modlin RL, Brightbill HD, Godowski PJ. The toll of innate immunity on microbial pathogens. N Engl J Med 1999;340:1834-1835.
17. Rogiers P. Hemofiltration treatment for sepsis: is it time for a controlled trial? Kidney Inter 1999;56:S99-S103.
18. Tetta C, Bellomo R, Brendolan A, Piccinni P, Digito A, Dan M, Irone M, Lonnemann G, Moscato D, Buades J, La Greca G, Ronco C. Use of adsorptive mechanisms in continuous renal replacement therapies in the critically ill. Kidney Inter 1999;56:S15-S19.
19. Liaudet L, Soriano FG, Szabo C. Biology of nitric oxide signaling. Crit Care Med 2000;28:N37-N52.
20. Thiemermann C. The use of selective inhibitors of inducible nitric oxide synthase in septic shock. Sepsis 1998;1:123-130.

21. Fischer SR, Bone HG, Harada M, Jourdain M, Traber D. Nitric oxide scavengers in sepsis. Sepsis 1998;1:137-144.
22. Creasey AA. New potential therapeutic modalities; tissue factor pathway inhibitor. Sepsis 1999;3:173-172.
23. Opal SM, Thijs LG. New potential therapeutic modalities; antithrombin III. Sepsis 1999;3:153-160.
24. Esmon CT. New potential therapeutic modalities; a PC. Sepsis 1999;3:161-172.
25. Czermak BJ, Sarma V, Pierson CL, Warner RL et al. Protective effects of C5a blockade in sepsis. Nature Med 1999;5:788-792.
26. Calandra T, Echtenacher B, Le Roy D, Pugin J, Metz CN, Hultner L, Heumann D, Mannel D, Bucala R, Glauser MP. Protection from septic shock by neutralization of macrophage migration inhibitory factor. Nature 2000;6:164-170.
27. Wang H, Bloom O, Zhang M, Vishnubhakat JM, Ombrellino M et al. HMG-1 as a late mediator of endotoxin lethality in mice. Science 1999;285;248-251.

Chapter 11

IMMUNOSTIMULATION IN SEPSIS

Hans-Dieter Volk, M.D., Ph.D., Kerstin Wolk, Ph.D; Robert Sabat, M.D., Wolf-Dietrich Döcke, M.D., Petra Reinke, M.D., Ph.D.
Institute of Medical Immunology and Department of Nephrology and Internal Intensive Medicine , Charité, Humboldt-University Berlin, Berlin, Germany

Introduction

Infectious complications remain a major problem in critically ill patients following trauma, burn injury, major surgery, or septic shock. The high risk of infection in these patients is related in part to the development of an acquired deficiency in host defense. Secondary infections can in turn result in sepsis which if severe is associated with a very high mortality. Over the last two decades our understanding of the pathophysiology of sepsis has progressed considerably. It is now clear that an overwhelming systemic inflammatory response to invasion by bacteria and fungi and/or their toxic products is important in the pathogenesis of SIRS, sepsis and multiple organ failure. Since TNF and IL-1 can mimic sepsis and septic shock in animal models, several recent clinical trials have focused on neutralization of these inflammatory mediators. These trials, however, have had very disappointing results.

Several reasons for the failure of the anti-inflammatory approach in sepsis have been proposed (1, 2). It is increasingly clear however that an assessment of immunological activity in individual patients may be essential for the rational use of immunomodulatory therapies. This is especially true in the critically ill patient in whom acquired immunosuppression may have resulted in infection and sepsis (3). In such patients, further inhibition of the host immune system may be harmful, while stimulation may actually be beneficial.

The beneficial effects of inflammatory mediators

During the past decade, many scientists (and companies) regarded TNF and IL-1 as the only 'bad guys' in sepsis despite the fact that experimental and clinical data were readily available contradicting this viewpoint. For example, TNF antagonists while successful in preventing shock following a bolus application of endotoxin (i.e. lipopolysaccharide, LPS) or bacteria in animals, showed no benefit or were even deleterious in the caecal ligation and puncture (CLP) peritonitis model which may be more relevant clinically (4). Moreover, mice genetically deficient in the production or response to TNF, while resistant to LPS mediated injury, were deficient in control of an infection due to live bacteria (5). This deficiency was associated with death even at low doses of live bacteria. Similar observations were made with lipopolysaccharide binding protein (LBP) knock out (k.o.) mice (6). On the other hand, mice deficient in anti-inflammatory cytokines, like TGF-ß or IL-10, are very sensitive to systemic inflammation related to LPS or bacterial challenge.

In light of this overall preclinical experience and the disappointing results in clinical trials of antiinflammatory therapies, we have come to understand that many of our animal models were too simple. An intravenous bolus of LPS or bacteria does not adequately reflect the complex host-pathogen interactions that take place during sepsis in humans. Furthermore, these data suggest that a well balanced inflammatory response is important for control of bacterial infections. Excessive inflammation in response to infection may be lethal just as too little inflammation may result in an uncontrolled spread of infection. While we appear to understand the mechanisms of shock, multiple organ failure and death induced by hyperinflammation, further studies are necessary to learn more about the pathogenesis of infection in models of 'hypoinflammation'. For example, we do not understand why the LBP -/- mice die from low dose Salmonella infection. Is the host's inflammatory system involved or does the bacteria play a direct toxic role?

Other types of clinical data also challenge the concept of septic death 'by too much inflammation'. For example, most patients with multiple organ failure due to sepsis have relatively low TNF plasma levels. Moreover, septic complications are more often observed in older patients and patients with advanced tumors, many of whom demonstrate a diminished immune responsiveness prior to the onset of sepsis.

Several groups including ours have reported deactivation of monocytes and granulocytes in septic patients, particularly during later stages of disease (3). In contrast to rapid and erratic fluctuations in serum cytokine concentrations, this cellular phenotype is remarkably stable. Whereas cytokines have half lives in plasma measured in minutes, monocytes and granulocytes, have a half-life in the peripheral blood of about 24 hrs. Monocytes migrate into the tissues where they differentiate into different subtypes of macrophages, whereas granulocytes continue to function, although for shorter periods after recruitment at sites of inflammation. The relative stability of circulating monocytes and neutrophils however make them suitable for daily monitoring.

In patients with prolonged sepsis we have demonstrated a state in which monocyte TNF secretion, HLA-DR antigen expression, and antigen-presenting capacity are all severely depressed. However, the ability of these cells to produce IL-1ra and, at least temporarly IL-10, is largely preserved. We noted that this switch to predominant anti-inflammatory mediator release by monocytes was associated with a high risk of fatal outcome from persistent infections which were in part opportunistic. In fact, none of the patients we monitored survived unless their monocytes recovered proinflammatory function and HLA-DR expression. This phenomenon which we initially observed in septic transplant patients, was termed 'immunoparalysis' (7, 8).

WHAT IS THE PATHOGENESIS OF 'IMMUNOPARALYSIS'?

Exogenous "overimmunosuppression"

Monocytes are a crucial component of resistance to infection. They phagocytize and kill pathogenic microorganisms, neutralize toxins originating from pathogens and as antigen-presenting cells and cytokine activated effector cells, are an important link between the innate resistance system and the highly specialized adaptive immune response. All of these functions are disturbed in monocytes from patients with 'immunoparalysis'.

The occurrence of 'immunoparalysis' does not appear to be related directly to invasion by specific pathogens or toxins. For example, we and others have observed monocyte deactivation and 'immunoparalysis' in some patients after sterile injury (burns, trauma, major surgery) or in the course of high-dose immunosuppression (7, 8). Thus, common host-derived regulatory processes may play an important role in this phenomenon. Monocyte phenotype and function are closely associated with the 'net'-immunosuppression of cell-mediated immunity, particularly of the type 1 T-cell response. The proinflammatory capacity of monocytes (secretion of TNF, IL-1, IL-12 etc.) as well their antigen-presenting capacity (expression of surface HLA-DR, HLA-DP, HLA-DQ, CD80/86) is positively regulated by immunostimulatory cytokines such as interferon-gamma [IFNγ] and GM-

CSF and negatively influenced by several factors including IL-10, TGF-ß, prostaglandins, catecholamines and apoptotic material.

Following high dose immunosuppression in transplant patients resulting from administration of a steroid bolus, OKT 3 mAb or ATG, we have seen a temporary decrease in both monocyte HLA-DR expression and capacity to generate TNF *ex vivo*. These decreases may be related to the lack of stimulatory cytokines such as IFNγ due to their downregulation by immunosuppression. In addition, steroids directly block cytokine action on monocytes and other cells while cyclosporine, another type of immunosuppressive agent, up-regulates monocyte TGF-ß secretion. In some patients monocyte deactivation may reach the level of 'immunoparalysis' – a situation which is associated with an increased risk of infection within several weeks. Indeed after two days of 'immunoparalysis', bacterial and/or fungal infections were seen in approximately 30 % of transplant patients vs. 4 % of patients without 'immunoparalysis'. The longer 'immunoparalysis' persists, the greater the incidence of infections (8). In general, immunocompetence rapidly recovers following reduction of immunosuppression. Several mechanisms in critically ill patients may result in 'immunoparalysis' similar to that associated with exogenous immunosuppression in transplant patients (Figure 1).

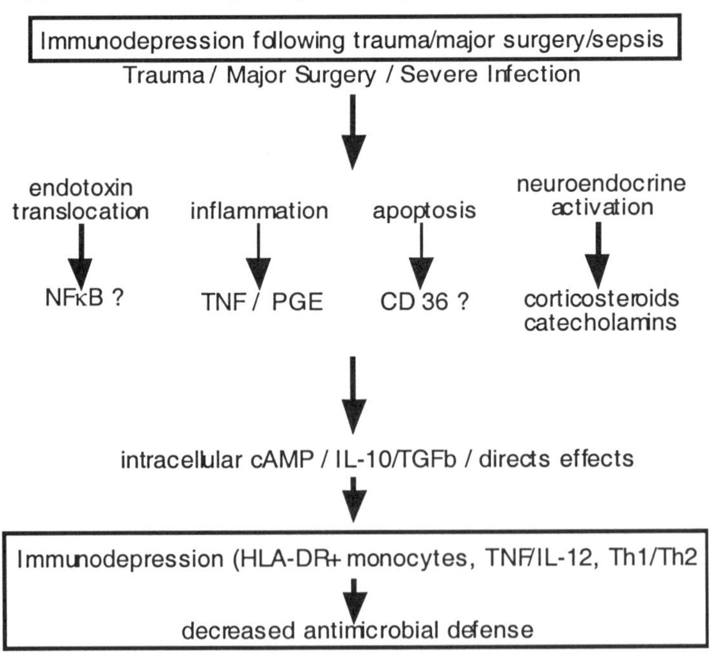

Figure 1. Mechanisms of monocyte deactivation: Inflammation, Apoptosis, and Stress

Role of IL-10 in 'immunoparalysis'

Almost all polytrauma, burn, or major surgery patients develop temporary monocyte deactivation within a few hours after the traumatic event. In some patients, this deactivation may be more severe (i.e. immunoparalysis) and long-lasting. Activation of the stress response may play an important role in downregulating systemic immune responsiveness in such patients. The regulatory role of the hypothalamic pituitary axis (HPA) controlling corticosteroid release is long established. Recently we have shown that activation of the catecholamine axis is also an important contributor to monocyte deactivation following stressful events. Studies on the molecular basis of this phenomenon revealed that cAMP dependent processes, including the up-regulation of IL-10, played a key role (Figure 1) (10). Experimental studies in rats supported interpretation of these clinical observations. Increased intracranial pressure or an intraventricular release of proinflammatory cytokines simulating head trauma, while not associated with systemic release of the pro-inflammatory cytokines TNF, IL-1, IFNγ or IL-6, both resulted in a rapid systemic release of the antiinflammatory cytokine IL-10, a drop in antigen-presenting activity, and diminished *ex vivo* TNF secretion capacity by peripheral blood and spleen monocyte/ macrophages (9). Concurrent inhibition of ß2-receptors prevented IL-10 release and monocyte/macrophage deactivation by 90 % and 50 %, respectively (9). Combined blockade of both stress pathways (ß2-adrenergic and steroid receptor blockade) almost completely prevented 'immunoparalysis' in this experimental model.

Following recovery both in ICU patients and in the rat model, monocyte/macrophage function returns spontaneously within 1-2 days following the stressful event. However, in some patients this downregulation of the immune response is more pronounced and long-lasting – a phenomenon that is associated with an increased risk of infection and sepsis, and poorer wound healing (e.g. anastomosis insufficiency). The phenomenon of long-lasting 'immunoparalysis' is seen in particular in patients with sepsis and septic shock.

What is different between patients with transient and long-lasting monocyte deactivation ?

Sepsis and sometimes major surgery and trauma are associated with endotoxemia related either to direct bacterial release or to translocation. Following *in vitro* LPS stimulation of blood leukocytes, TNF secretion peaks about 2 hrs later whereas peak secretion of IL-10 requires more than 14 hrs.

TNF by itself can upregulate IL-10 expression. A high concentration of TNF leads to hyperinflammation but at the same time also induces IL-10 which will tend to downregulate the inflammatory reaction. In fact, *in vitro* treatment of monocytes with IL-10 reduces their HLA-DR expression, antigen-presenting activity, and TNF secretion while the IL-1RA secretion is increased – a phenotype quite similar to the 'immunoparalysis' phenomenon. Moreover, neutralisation of IL-10 blocks LPS desensitisation, a phenomenon in which monocyte TNF release is inhibited by a prior exposure to a low dose of LPS (3, 10). These data suggest that inflammation by itself may induce its own downregulation via the NFkB pathway induced by TNF (Figure 1). The monocyte deactivation frequently observed in patients surviving septic shock (late sepsis) may be related to this phenomenon of counter-regulation, termed 'CARS' by Dr. Roger Bone (11).

Inflammation and infection are frequently associated with apoptotic cell death. In order to prevent overwhelming inflammation, scavenging apoptotic material by monocytes itself downregulates TNF secretion and upregulates IL-10 secretion (Figure 1). The molecular mechanism underlying this is not fully understood but CD14/CD36 receptors seem to be involved. A massive induction of apoptosis in organ failure (e.g. liver failure) may contribute to the phenomenon of 'immunoparalysis' in septic and trauma patients.

Moreover, the stress axis seems to also be involved in the regulation of IL-10 released during systemic inflammation and infection. In contrast to the situation *in vitro*, in both humans and mice, TNF and IL-10 are secreted in parallel within one hour following LPS challenge suggesting the involvement of TNF-independent mechanisms for IL-10 regulation. Using RT-PCR analyses we found very high TNF and IL-10 mRNA expression in mouse or rat livers 1 hour after LPS injection while peripheral blood leukocytes expressed TNF only. Eight hours later, IL-10 mRNA was also detectable in blood leukocytes and the protein product was, in contrast to TNF, still detectable in the plasma. Both late IL-10 mRNA and IL-10 protein expression were inhibited by the application of a neutralizing anti-TNF mAb in parallel with LPS. In contrast, early IL-10 synthesis was not reduced following inhibition of TNF. However, with ß2-adrenergic receptor blockade not only was early IL-10 release strongly inhibited but early TNF release was increased (Volk et al., in preparation).

In summary, IL-10 is induced by different pathways (stress response, uptake of apoptotic material, and inflammation) (12). Similar effects in combination may explain the more long-lasting 'immunoparalysis' seen in patients with LPS translocation after severe trauma/major surgery or during sepsis. However, other data suggests that IL-10 is not the only important mediator in this regard.

IL-10 is not the complete story of "immunoparalysis"

Compared to normal controls, plasma samples from patients with monocyte deactivation following major surgery or in septic patients inhibited monocyte HLA-DR expression and *ex vivo* TNF secretion by cells from healthy donors. In most samples, elevated IL-10 levels were detectable but the differences between the patients that did and did not develop 'immunoparalysis' were only marginal. Neutralizing IL-10 mAb showed variable effects in that it abolished the inhibitory activity of the plasma samples by 20 to 100 %. This suggests that additional immunosuppressive factors may have been present (Syrbe et al., submitted). Moreover, we recently performed a clinical trial in which IL-10 was used for treatment of psoriasis. The patients received subcutaneous IL-10 in daily doses up to 12 μg/kg b.w. for several weeks resulting in plasma IL-10 levels comparable with those seen in many ICU patients (20-100 pg/ml). As expected, monocyte HLA-DR expression, antigen-presenting activity, *ex vivo* TNF/IL-12 secretion capacity, and the Th1-/Th2- cytokine ratio were significantly inhibited (13). Despite administration of IL-10 however, monocyte downregulation was not as great as that seen with 'immunoparalysis'. Again, this suggests that while IL-10 is an important player in monocyte deactivation, it is not the only one. As long-lasting immunosuppression in ICU patients is frequently associated with endotoxemia related to either systemic infection or translocation, we wondered whether endotoxin itself could contribute to the pathogenesis of 'immunoparalysis'. Very recently we compared monocyte deactivation following endotoxin priming (simulation of endotoxemia) and IL-10 treatment (simulation of stress response only). Our data indicated that endotoxin mediates its suppressive effects mainly via IL-10 but provokes a more profound and longer-lasting antiinflammatory state in monocytes than IL-10 does alone, suggesting additional co-factors which maintain the IL-10 induced monocyte deactivation in patients with endotoxemia (14).

In addition the patient's predisposition is a further factor which clearly has a major impact on the balance between inflammation and anti-inflammation. Allelic polymorphism's have been described which are associated with low or high IL10 and TNF production, respectively (15).

HOW CAN WE RESTORE IMMUNE RESPONSIVENESS?

Tapering down exogenous immunosuppression

If 'immunoparalysis' is not just an epiphenomenon but is in fact causally related to an increased incidence of infection and to a poor prognosis in septic patients, then promoting recovery from immunodeficiency should be a useful therapeutic approach. The first evidence that this may be a feasible concept came from transplant patients. In patients undergoing high-dose immunosuppression as induction or anti-rejection therapy we monitor monocyte function two to three times per week. HLA-DR expression is determined by flowcytometry. In the patients 'overimmunosuppression', defined as < 30 % HLA-DR+ monocytes (with the new quantitative method: < 5000 molecules/cell), is associated with a 7.5 fold increased risk of infection within the next two to three weeks. In such cases we now reduce the immunosuppression carefully and additionally monitor the patient in order to quickly detect incipient infections. This decreased the incidence of severe infections in our transplant population.

If 'immunoparalysis' is observed in transplant patients with established infections, we immediately taper down immunosuppression in order to prevent death by sepsis. With one exception, we have never seen acute graft rejection as a result of reducing immunosuppression in patients with 'immunoparalysis', underscoring the general nature of the immunodeficiency in these patients. In sharp contrast, reduction of immunosuppression in infected transplant patients without 'immunoparalysis' is frequently followed by acute rejection (7, 8). In summary, the transplant data suggest that the recovery of an inflammatory response is important for the control of bacterial/fungal infections and that it is not harmful even in septic patients. These observations were the rational for similar approaches in non-transplant septic patients.

IFNγ treatment

In vitro, ex vivo and in animal models, we first showed that the monocytic activators IFNγ and GM-CSF were able to reverse the state of monocyte deactivation (16, 17). Moreover, we demonstrated in a pilot trial that IFNγ can also reverse 'immunoparalysis' in septic patients *in vivo* (3). This was the first trial of a therapeutic intervention strategy in sepsis which used immune monitoring parameters as a guideline for treatment. Nine septic patients with 'immunoparalysis', defined as <30% HLA-DR+ monocytes persisting for at least two days, were treated every day with 100 μg/d IFNγ s.c.. Treatment was continued until more than 50 % of monocytes were HLA-DR+ for three consecutive days (duration of treatment: mean 6 days, range 4 to 11 days). Although IFNγ dramatically increases LPS related mortality in animal sepsis models, it was well tolerated by the patients with 'immunoparalysis'. Furthermore, while the kinetics and the level of the response varied from individual to individual, monocyte recovery was observed in all nine patients (3). The slightly upregulated TNF plasma levels (23 pg/ml peak level on day 4, vs. 4 pg/ml before therapy) reflected the restoration of monocyte function *in vivo* and the recovery of an antimicrobial response. Eight of nine patients recovered from sepsis shortly after treatment, although two of them relapsed at a later stage when IFNγ treatment was discontinued. In parallel, the MOF score improved significantly. This pilot trial was not designed to prove effects on mortality but the results were promising.

G-CSF treatment

Several groups have reported diminished granulocyte function in septic patients. Also, monocytes from patients with 'immunoparalysis' had a diminished capacity to secrete G-CSF. As G-CSF is not only important for granulocytopoesis but also for the antimicrobial function of mature granulocytes, we wondered whether G-CSF application would be a therapeutic alternative in sepsis. Twelve septic patients (abdominal/thoracic sepsis; three with ARDS) who had 'immunoparalysis' for at least two days were treated with G-CSF (3x300 μg) despite leukocytosis (mean 13 GPT/l). No significant side effects were observed. Leukocyte counts increased up to 75 GPT/l (mean 35 GPT/l) in 10/12 patients. Nine of them recovered from sepsis and this was associated with a decrease in procalcitonin plasma levels (Zuckermann et al., in preparation).

Plasmapheresis for removal of suppressive plasma factors

In another approach we tested the effectiveness of plasmapheresis in septic patients with 'immunoparalysis'. The rationale for this therapy is the removal of inhibitory factors from the plasma which cannot be achieved by dialysis. For this pilot trial we took 76 septic patients with 'immunoparalysis' for more than 4 days. 35 of them underwent plasmapheresis (3x 4-5 l). Eighteen of these 35 patients responded with stable recovery of monocyte function. Seventeen of the 18 responders survived but none of the 17 non-responders did. Overall mortality was 52 % with treatment versus 80 % in the untreated control group ($p<0.01$) (8, 18).

CONCLUSIONS

The immune system should be regarded as an organ which in ICU patients can be driven to failure just as a liver or a kidney can. The monitoring of function in other systems (kidney, liver, blood pressure, lung, coagulation etc.) is well established in ICUs, but monitoring of the immune system is still poorly developed. However, immune responsiveness is essential for the control of infections. In this sense the failure of immunotherapeutic approaches in sepsis introduced without immune monitoring may not be surprising. The data from our pilot trials suggest that immunostimulation in septic patients with defined 'immunoparalysis' may provide a novel therapeutic approach. Controlled multicenter trials will be necessary to test this hypothesis. In the past, poor standardization of immune monitoring made multicenter trials very difficult. However, this problem has been largely obviated by the recent development of well standardized tests for immune parameters. On the one hand immune competence can be measured by a quantitative HLA-DR flow cytometric measurement and by a semi-automatic *ex vivo* whole blood TNF secretion assay, while on the other hand inflammation and tissue injury can be detected by measurement of plasma TNF and IL-6 levels by semiautomatic systems (19). Moreover, it has been shown that measurement of procalcitonin plasma levels is helpful for early detection and monitoring of invasive bacterial/fungal infections (Figure 2).

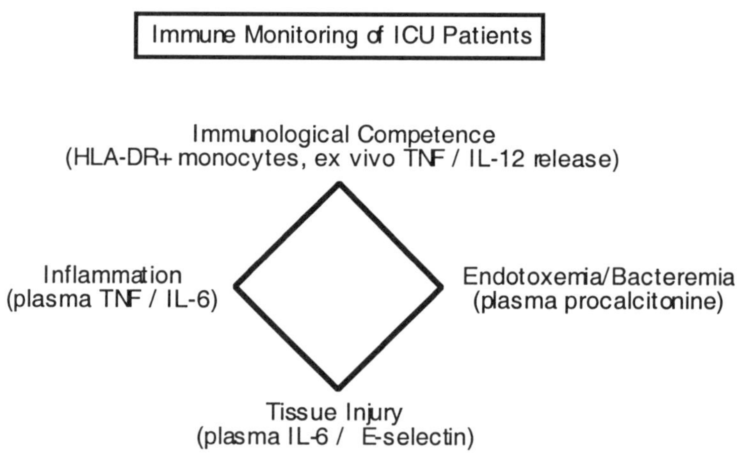

Figure 2. Recommendations for differential immune monitoring in ICU patients

In our view, preemptive therapy of high-risk patients would be a much better approach than the treatment of established sepsis. In order to improve the cost/benefit ratio of immune interventions measurement of immunocompetence, such as monocytic HLA-DR expression or whole blood TNF/IL-12 release, may help to detect patients at high risk of developing infectious complications after major surgery and trauma. After an initial downregulation of the monocytic system which is seen in almost all patients after major surgery and trauma, immune function recovers in most patients, while long-lasting immune deactivation is associated with an increased risk in development of infection. By day 2 of postoperative immunodepression, the positive predictive value is already >90 %. It should therefore be possible to accurately select the high risk patients who may benefit from a preemptive immunostimulatory therapy. With the availability of standardised immune monitoring procedures we can now design appropriate clinical trials.

Acknowlegement: This work was supported by DFG (SFB 421)

REFERENCES

1. Natanson C, Hoffman WD, Suffredini AF, Eichacker PQ, Danner RL. Selected treatment strategies for septic shock based on proposed mechanisms of pathogenesis. Ann Intern Med 1994; 120: 771-783.
2. Zeni F, Freeman B, Natanson C. Anti-inflammatory therapies to treat sepsis and septic shock: a reassessment. Crit Care Med 1997; 25: 1095-1100.
3. Döcke WD, Randow F, Syrbe U, Krausch D, Asadullah K, Reinke P, Volk HD, Kox W . Monocyte deactivation in septic patients: restoration by IFN-γ treatment. Nature Med 1997; 3: 678-681.
4. Echtenacher B, Falk W, Mannel DN, Krammer PH. Requirement of endogenous tumor necrosis factor/cachectin for recovery from experimental peritonitis. J Immunol 1990; 145: 3762-3766.
5. Pfeffer K. Mice deficient for the p55 kD tumor necrosis factor receptor are resistant to endotoxic shock, yet succumb to L. monocytogenes infection. Cell 1993; 73: 457-467.
6. Jack RS, Fan X, Bernheiden M, Rune G, Ehlers M, Weber A, Kirsch G, Mentel R, Fürll B, Freudenberg M, Schmitz G, Stelter F, Schütt C. Lipopolysaccaride binding protein is required to combat a murine gram-negative bacterial infection. Nature 1997; 389: 742-745.
7. Volk HD, Reinke P, Falck P Staffa G, Briedigkeit H, von Baehr R. Diagnostic value of an immune monitoring program for the clinical management of immunosuppressed patients with septic complications. Clin Transplant 1989; 3: 246-252.
8. Döcke WD, Reinke P, Syrbe U, Platzer C, Asadullah K, Krausch D, Zuckermann H, Volk HD. Immunoparalysis in sepsis – from phenomenon to treatment strategies. Transplantationsmedizin 1997; 9: 55-65.
9. Woiciechowsky C, Asadullah K, Nestler D, Eberhardt B, Platzer C, Schöning B, Glöckner F, Lanksch WR, Volk HD, Döcke WD. Sympathetic activation triggers systemic IL-10 release in immunodepression induced by brain injury. Nature Med 1998; 4: 808-813.
10. Randow F, Syrbe U, Meisel C, Krausch D, Zuckermann H, Platzer C, Volk HD. Mechanism of endotoxin desensitization – involvement of IL-10 and TGFß. J Exp Med 1995; 5: 1887-1892.
11. Bone RC. Sir Isaac Newton, sepsis, SIRS, CARS. Crit Care Med 1996; 24:1125-8.

12. van Dissel J, van Langevelde P, Westendorp RG, Kwappenberg K, Frolich M. Anti-inflammatory cytokine profile and mortality in febrile patients. Lancet 1998; 351: 950-953.
13. Asadullah K, Stephanek K, Leupold M, Jasulaitis D, Audring H, Volk HD, Sterry W, Döcke WD. IL-10 is a key cytokine in psoriasis. Proof of principle by IL-10 therapy: a new therapeutic approach. J Clin Invest 1998; 101: 1-12.
14. Wolk K, Döcke WD, v.Baehr V, Volk HD, Sabat R. Impaired antigen presentation by human monocytes during endotoxin tolerance. Blood 2000; in press.
15. Eskdale J, Gallagher G, Verweij CL, Keijsers V, Westendorp RG, Huizinga TW. Interleukin 10 secretion in relation to human IL-10 locus haplotypes. Proc Natl Acad Sci USA 1998; 95: 9465-9470.
16. Randow F, Randow F, Döcke WD, Bundschuh DS, Hartung T, Wendel A, Volk HD. In vitro prevention and reversal of LPS desensitization by IFNg, IL-12, and GM-CSF. J Immunol 1997; 158: 2911-2918.
17. Bundschuh D, Barsig J, Hartung T, Randow F, Döcke WD, Volk HD, Wendel A. GM-CSF and interferon-gamma restore the systemic TNFalpha response to endotoxin in lipopolysaccaride-desensitized mice. J Immunol 1997; 158: 2862-2871.
18. Reinke P. Plasmapheresis in the therapy of septic disease. Int J Artif Organs 1997; 19: 127-128.
19. Reinke P, Döcke WD, Kox W, Zuckermann H, Volk HD. New trends in immune monitoring of ICU patients. Dtsch Med Wschr 1999; 124: 1527-30.

Chapter 12

GRANULOCYTE COLONY STIMULATING FACTOR AS A THERAPY FOR PNEUMONIA AND SEPSIS IN THE NONNEUTROPENIC HOST: PRECLINICAL AND CLINICAL TRIALS

Chantal Parent, D.V.M. and Peter Q. Eichacker, M.D.
Critical Care Medicine Department, Clinical Center National Institutes of Health, Bethesda, MD 20892

Introduction

Outcome associated with severe pneumonia, especially when it is complicated by sepsis and septic shock remains poor in the nonneutropenic host despite our best conventional therapies (30 to 50%) (1,2). New modes of therapy are needed. An alternative to blocking the intense inflammatory response of sepsis, an approach which has not shown convincing benefit in clinical trials thus far, is to administer agents to augment host defense and better control the underlying infection. One such agent is recombinant granulocyte colony stimulating factor (G-CSF), a potent stimulator of neutrophil number and function (3,4). Similar to antiinflammatory agents however, despite promising results in preclinical studies, G-CSF has not shown convincing benefit in early clinical trials in nonneutropenic patients presenting with pneumonia or sepsis (5,6). While disappointing, our evolving preclinical and clinical experience with G-CSF may provide insight into ways to increase the effectiveness of this therapeutic approach in the future.

From the outset, there was concern regarding the potential effects of neutrophil stimulation with G-CSF in nonneutropenic patients with severe infection. Data both in animal models and patients had implicated the neutrophil in the pathogenesis of sepsis induced tissue injury (1). This was most notable in the lung, where the neutrophil had been strongly associated with the development of the acute respiratory distress syndrome (ARDS) during pneumonia and sepsis. However, several lines of evidence supported the use of G-CSF in severe infection. The neutrophil is an early cellular component in the phagocytosis and clearance of microbes and microbial toxins at sites of bacterial infection. Abnormalities of neutrophil function increase the risk and severity of infection and sepsis. Reductions in endogenous G-CSF had been shown to cause abnormalities of neutrophil number and function (7,8). Finally, administration of G-CSF decreased the risk of infection in neutropenic animals and humans (3,4).

Early studies in nonneutropenic animals suggested that G-CSF would be beneficial and not harmful during severe infection. In different small animal models including several with intrapulmonary infection, G-CSF most often administered before infectious challenge, increased survival (9-12). Other early preclinical studies showed that pretreatment with G-CSF did not worsen nonpulmonary or pulmonary injury in nonneutropenic animals challenged with intravenous endotoxin (13-15). Endotoxin is a microbial toxin which has been closely associated with stimulation of neutrophil mediated inflammatory tissue injury. Based on these preclinical findings, clinical studies with G-CSF were initiated in nonneutropenic patients with severe infection or sepsis. In contrast to many early animal studies however, in most clinical studies G-CSF was administered therapeutically, following the onset of infection.

Clinical Experience with G-CSF Therapy in Pneumonia and Sepsis

Early phase 1 trials testing the effects of G-CSF in nonneutropenic patients presenting with pneumonia or other severe infections suggested that it was safe (16-19). DeBoisblanc et al administered G-CSF in daily doses ranging from 75 to 600 μg in a total of 30 patients presenting with community acquired pneumonia (CAP) (16). None of these patients died or developed clinically evident pulmonary complications related to G-CSF. Hustinix et al. found that survival in 10 patients with severe ventilator dependent pneumonia was greater with G-CSF administration than would have been predicted by APACHE-II scoring (i.e. 70% observed versus 40% predicted) (17). Endo et al. administered G-CSF to 24 patients in which severe sepsis had resulted in relative reductions in circulating neutrophils (18). Although neutrophil counts increased in all 19 survivors shortly after the start of G-CSF, they remained low in the 5 nonsurvivors until death. There was no evident toxicity with G-CSF in patients that survived. Finally, in a study by Gross-Weege et al. administration of G-CSF in a group of 20 postoperative surgical patients increased neutrophil counts greater in the 10 with the systemic inflammatory response syndrome (SIRS) without evidence of infection compared to 10 with sepsis and documented infection (19). All 10 patients with SIRS but only 6 of 10 with sepsis survived. Overall, absence of evident toxicity in these phase 1 trials supported continued investigation with G-CSF in noneutropenic patients. Of interest however were the possibly reduced or absent effects of therapeutic G-CSF on circulating neutrophil numbers in patients with more severe sepsis and a higher likelihood of dying (18,19).

Two nonrandomized phase 2 trials compared the effects of therapeutic G-CSF in critically ill patients to historical control patients. Ishikawa et. al. administered G-CSF to septic patients meeting 3 criteria: (1) sepsis according to the criteria of the American College of Chest Physicians and the Society of Critical Care Medicine, (2) relative neutropenia with a total circulating leukocyte count less than 5,000/mm^3, and (3) a serum concentration of C-reactive protein of more than 10 mg/dl (20). Patients admitted to their institution in the recent past meeting similar criteria served as controls. In this study, G-CSF increased survival (17 of 23 with G-CSF versus 8 of 19 controls, $p=0.09$) and circulating neutrophil numbers and function and reduced CRP, IL-6 and IL-8 levels and APACHE-II scores. Nishida et al. studied the effects of G-CSF in patients with relative neutropenia related to sepsis following gastrointestinal perforation (21). Compared to historical controls, patients receiving therapeutic G-CSF had better survival (6 of 8 with G-CSF versus 8 of 23 controls, $p<0.08$) and increases in circulating neutrophil counts and decreases in organ injury. Thus, these small nonrandomized phase 2 trials suggested that G-CSF was not only safe but might also be beneficial in nonneutropenic critically ill patients.

Based on early preclinical and phase 1 and nonrandomized phase 2 trials, prospective randomized trials were initiated assessing the effects of G-CSF treatment in patients presenting with severe pneumonia. In a phase 2 study in patients with pneumonia and sepsis, Wunderink et al. showed that G-CSF was associated with trends towards increased survival (2 of 6 control versus 9 of 12 G-CSF patients, $p=0.11$) and better resolution of organ injury (23). There was no apparent pulmonary toxicity associated with G-CSF. In the first published phase 3 trial with G-CSF in noneutropenic subjects, Nelson et al. administered it to patients presenting with CAP in association with 1 of 7 risk factors (Table 1) (5). Overall survival was high in the study and did not differ between treatment groups (357 of 380 with G-CSF versus 352 of 376 controls). G-CSF was associated with significant increases in circulating neutrophils but did not alter the time to resolution of morbidity, a composite score which was the primary end point of the study (Table 2). However, time to resolution of chest radiographic abnormalities, a component in the score, was shorter with G-CSF ($p=0.03$). Furthermore, several complications, including empyema, ARDS and disseminated intravascular coagulation, were reported to be reduced with G-CSF. In a subgroup analysis of patients presenting with multi-lobar infiltrates, G-CSF was reported to be associated with a significant reduction in the primary endpoint ($p=0.045$) and a trend towards increased survival (128 of 138 with G-CSF versus 108 of 123 controls, p=0.18).

Table 1. Risk Factors for Inclusion of Patients with Community Acquired Pneumonia into a Phase 3 Study with Therapeutic G-CSF

Age greater than 65 years
Preexisting chronic illness involving the heart, lung or kidneys
Splenectomy
Multilobar infitrates on chest radiograph
Relative leukopenia (i.e. leukocytes less than 6,000/mm^3)
Hypoxemia
Transient hypotension

Revised from Nelson et al., JID 1998

Table 2. Definition of the Time to Resolution of Morbidity Score in a Phase 3 Study of Therapeutic G-CSF in Patients with Community Acquired Pneumonia

Number of days between randomization and the first day when all the following occurred:
Improvement or stability of all abnormalities on chest radiograph by comparison with previous serial films
Respiratory rate ≤ 24 breaths/min for 24 h
Oral temparature ≤37.9 for 24 h
Normalized oxygenation, defined as a PaO2/FiO2 ≥285 OR ≥90% O2 saturation on room air. For patients with prior hypoxemia, a return to within 10% of the most recent prepneumonia PaO2/FiO2 was required.

Revised from Nelson et al., JID 1998

In order to confirm what appeared to be potentially beneficial effects with G-CSF in intial randomized phase 2 and 3 trials in patients with CAP and multilobar infitrates or with pneumonia and sepsis, 2 subsequent phase 3 trials were conducted. Preliminary reports are available from both of these studies (6). Despite studying a much larger number of patients (N=480) with CAP and multilobar infiltrates however, G-CSF was still not associated with significant increases in survival (92% with G-CSF versus 88% in controls, p=0.18). Subgroup analysis in that study has suggested that G-CSF was beneficial in patients with pneumococcal pneumonia (92% survival with G-CSF versus 77% in controls, p=0.07) however this requires confirmation. In a phase 3 trial in patients (N=700) with pneumonia and sepsis, in contrast to the phase 2 trial, G-CSF was associated with a small reduction in survival, although this was not significant (71% with G-CSF versus 75% in controls, p=0.22). While also not significant there was an increased incidence of ARDS in patients receiving G-CSF in this trial (11% with G-CSF versus 6% in controls).

In summary then, despite promising results in early preclinical and phase 1 and 2 clinical trials, in phase 3 trials treatment with G-CSF in nonneutropenic patients presenting with severe pneumonia, have been varied and overall appear negligible (Fig. 1). These inconsistent results with G-CSF suggest that factors capable of influencing the effects of G-CSF may have differed among both these preclinical and clinical trials. More recent preclinical studies have identified several such factors.

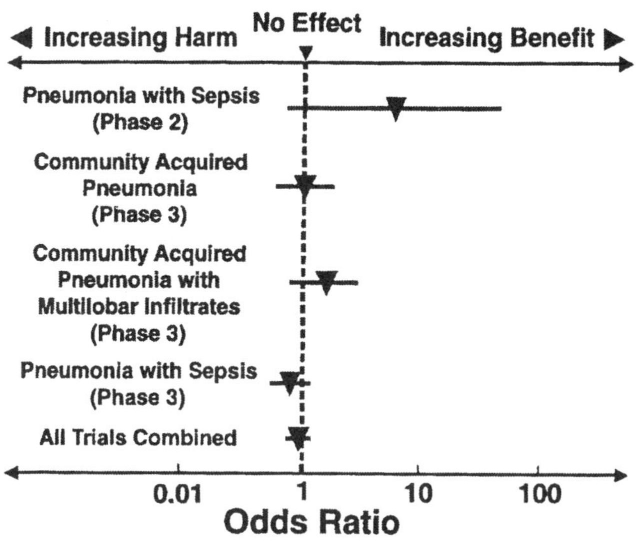

Figure 1. The effect of G-CSF on the odds ratio of survival (inverted triangles) and ther 95% confidence interval for these effects (horizontal bars) in 4 randomized phase 2 or 3 trials in nonneutropenic patients with pneumonia. G-CSF did not change the odds ratio of survival significantly in any of these trials and its overall effects (bottom odds ratio) in the trials was negligible.

Factors Potentially Influencing the Effects of G-CSF Therapy

One factor potentially altering the effects of G-CSF is the timing of therapy. In contrast to prophylactic administration, as used in many early preclinical models, therapeutic G-CSF administered after the onset of infection similar to clinical trials with pneumonia and sepsis may contribute little to an already stimulated host defense response in the nonneutropenic patient. Data from several studies support this possibility. In canines, we found that prophylactic treatment with 12 daily doses of G-CSF (5ug/kg) starting 9 d before intraperitoneal inoculation with an *E. coli* infected thrombin-fibrin clot and initiation of antibiotic therapy, was very beneficial (24). Compared to controls, G-CSF increased circulating neutrophils both before and following the onset of sepsis, decreased blood bacteria, endotoxin and tumor necrosis factors levels and improved hemodynamic function and survival (Fig. 2 and 3). Importantly, lung neutrophil accumulation and injury associated with sepsis in this model were not worsened with G-CSF. In order to then test the effectiveness of therapeutic G-CSF, in a subsequent study using this same model, we administered G-CSF or placebo in several different doses comparable to or greater than the total doses given prophylactically but started after *E. coli* inoculation (25). Therapeutic G-CSF given to uninfected animals receiving sterile clot caused rapid dose ordered increases in circulating neutrophil numbers and no harmful effects. In *E. coli* infected animals with sepsis however, therapeutic G-CSF resulted in paradoxical dose ordered reductions in circulating neutrophils and worsened hemodynamic function and survival. Of note, we had shown previously that the onset of sepsis in this model was associated with high endogenous G-CSF levels which may have negated the effects of exogenous therapeutic G-CSF (26). Overall in other published animal models of infection with antibiotic support, G-CSF appeared to result in more pronounced beneficial effects on survival when given prophylactically than therapeutically (11, 27-33). In clinical studies, prophylactic treatment with G-CSF in patients was associated with reductions in the incidence of sepsis or bacteremia in two small prospective randomized studies (34, 35). However, overall survival was high in these studies and reductions in infection with G-CSF were not associated with measurable improvements in outcome.

Factors having to do with bacterial infection itself may also alter the effects of G-CSF. Following our study showing that prophylactic G-CSF improved survival without altering lung injury in peritonitis, we tested a similar regimen in canines challenged with intrabronchial *E. coli* to simulate bacterial pneumonia (36). As with peritonitis, G-CSF increased circulating neutrophils both before and following the onset of sepsis, decreased blood endotoxin and tumor necrosis factors levels and improved hemodynamic function and survival. In contrast to peritonitis however, this regimen of G-CSF worsened lung injury as reflected by changes in arterial oxygenation. Thus the site of infection appeared to alter the potentially harmful inflammatory effects of G-CSF. In this canine model however, G-CSFs beneficial effect on host defense appeared to outweigh its potentially harmful effects on lung injury. In a subsequent study though in rats challenged with a dose of intrabronchial *E. coli* 4 fold greater than the one given to canines, G-CSF not only increased lung neutrophils and injury but also worsened survival (Fig. 4 and 5). Thus in this study it appeared that G-CSFs effect on inflammatory lung injury had negated its beneficial host defense effect (37).

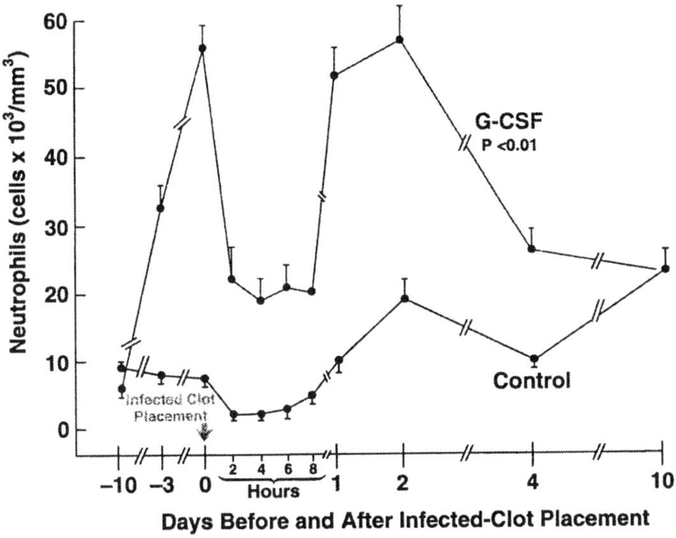

Figure 2. Serial mean (± SEM) circulating neutrophil numbers, at baseline before and following initiation of a 12 d regimen of G-CSF or placebo (control) started 8 d before surgical intraperitoneal placement of an *E. coli* infected thrombin-fibrin clot.

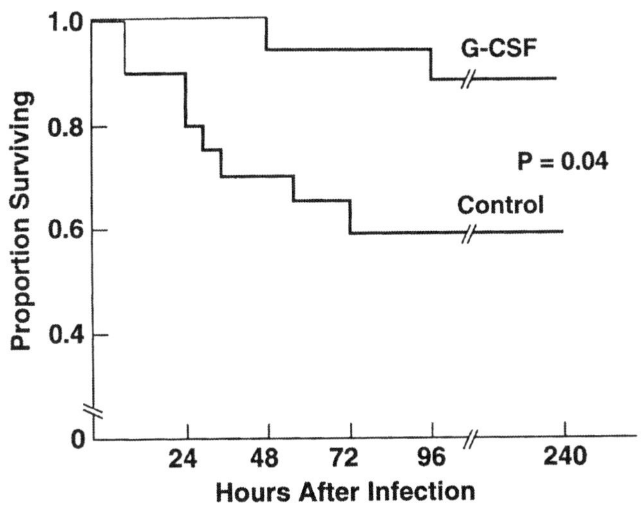

Figure 3. Proportion of animals surviving with prophylactic G-CSF or placebo (control) versus time (h) following surgical intraperitoneal placement of an *E. coli* infected thrombin-fibrin clot.

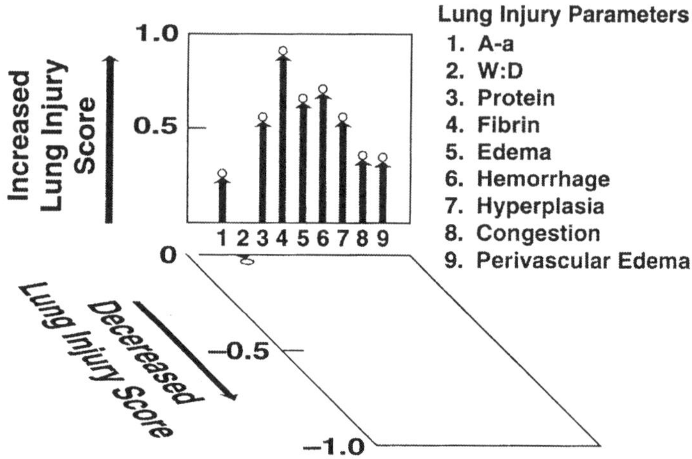

Figure 4. Lung injury score for 9 parameters of lung injury shown on the right of the figure for rats treated with G-CSF before and following intrabronchial inoculation with *E. coli*. Positive and negative scores represent mean differences in lung injury compared with control animals. Upward-pointing arrows represent increased lung injury compared with control animals. Following the onset of pneumonia G-CSF was associated with increases in 8 of 9 parameters of lung injury in a pattern that was very significant (p<0.001). Lung injury was assessed 6 to 12 hs following inoculation.

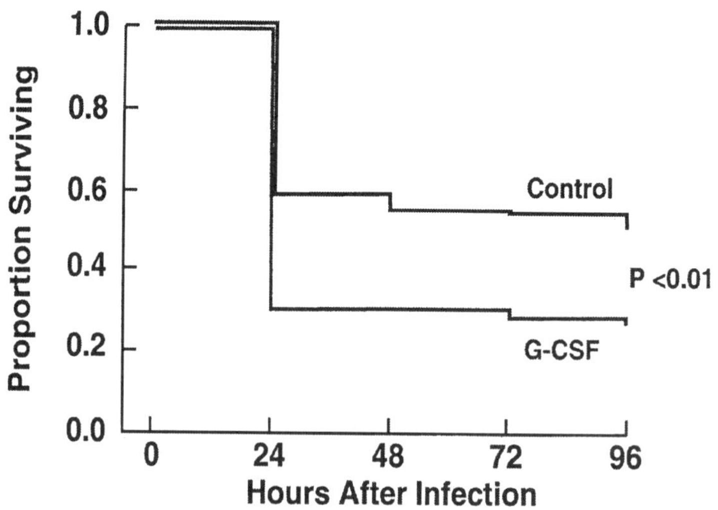

Figure 5. Proportion of animals surviving with G-CSF or placebo (control) versus time (h) following intrabronchial inoculation with *E. coli*.

In contrast to our findings with *E. coli* pneumonia in rats, several early studies had shown that G-CSF treatment increased survival with pulmonary infection related to either *S.pneumoniae* or *K. pneumoniae* (9,12,38). In combination these studies suggested that type of bacterial infection might also alter the effects of G-CSF. To test this possibility, in collaboration with Dr. Waheed Karzai, we compared the effects of treatment with G-CSF in rats challenged with similarly lethal intrabronchial doses of either *E. coli* or *S. aureus.* (38). With *E. coli* challenge, G-CSF caused paradoxical reductions in circulating neutrophils and, as we had seen previously, worsened lung injury and survival (Figure 6). In a pattern that was very different, with *S. aureus* pneumonia, G-CSF increased circulating neutrophils and improved survival. These findings suggested that microbial or host mediators associated with *E. coli* but not *S. aureus* infection were capable of interacting with G-CSF stimulated circulating neutrophils to cause increased clearance of these cells and worsened host defense or inflammatory tissue injury.

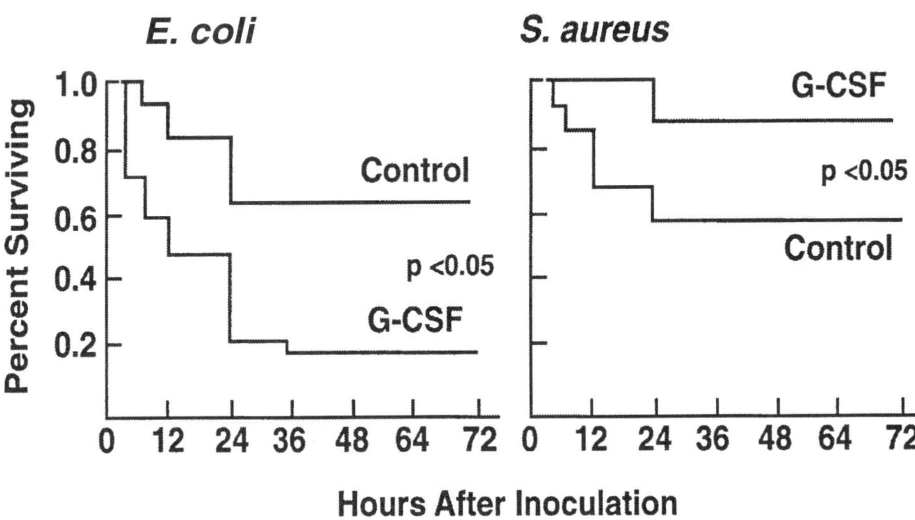

Figure 6. Proportion of animals surviving with G-CSF or placebo (control) versus time (h) following intrabronchial inoculation with *E. coli* (Panel A) or *S. aureus* (Panel B).

A final factor with the potential to influence the effects of G-CSF during pneumonia, relates to the presence or absence of concurrent therapies. Patients with severe pneumonia frequently require mechanical ventilation and oxygen support. Both these therapies have been associated with neutrophil mediated lung injury related to either barotrauma or to oxygen toxicity which independent of infection could be aggravated during treatment with G-CSF. In support of this, in rats, treatment with G-CSF aggravated lung injury related to increased inspired oxygen concentrations (Figure 7) (37). Furthermore, treatment with G-CSF worsened lung injury and survival in rats ventilated with tidal volumes associated with high distending airway pressures and barotrauma (40).

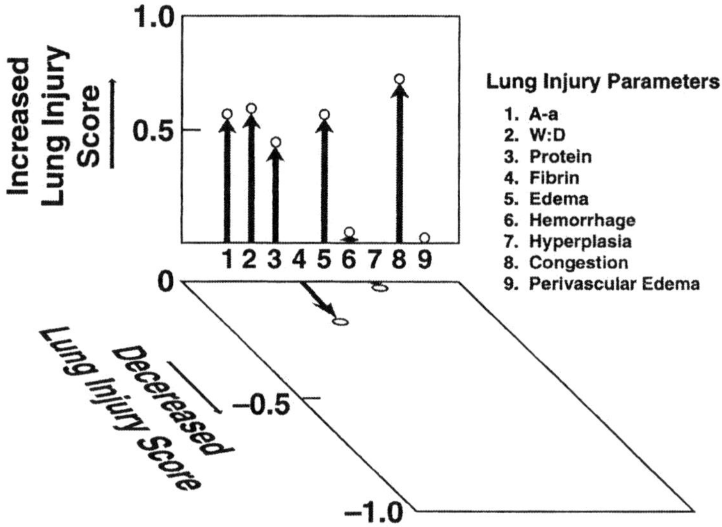

Figure 7. Lung injury score for 9 parameters of lung injury shown on the right of the figure for rats treated with G-CSF before and following exposure to lethal hyperoxia (fractional inspired oxygen concentration 0.90). Positive and negative scores represent mean differences in lung injury compared with control animals. Upward-pointing arrows represent increased lung injury compared with control animals. Following the onset of pneumonia G-CSF was associated with increases in 8 of 9 parameters of lung injury in a pattern that was very significant ($p<0.001$). Lung injury was assessed 96hs following initiation of hyperoxia.

Conclusions

Thus, preclinical studies indicate that factors like timing of therapy, site and type of bacterial infection and development of noninfectious lung injury may alter the effects of G-CSF during severe infection and sepsis. These studies suggest that G-CSF may be most beneficial in nonneutropenic patients if used prophylactically in those at high risk of infection. However, these studies also suggest that neutrophil stimulation with G-CSF during the development of severe pneumonia and sepsis may be associated with adverse effects with some bacterial types and when the risk of neutrophil mediated lung injury of noninfectious causes is high. Variation in factors such as these may in part explain the inconsistent effects noted with G-CSF therapy in preclinical and clinical trials. Despite disappointing results in early randomized clinical trials testing G-CSF, augmenting host defense is still a promising therapeutic approach for patients with or at risk of severe infection and sepsis. This approach however continues to require research to determine in which patients and under what conditions it will be most effective (41).

REFERENCES

1. Natanson C, Hoffman WD, Suffredini AF, Eichacker PQ, Danner RL. Selected treatment strategies for septic shock based on proposed mechanisms of pathogenesis. Ann Intern Med 1994;120(9):771-783.
2. Freeman B, Eichacker PQ, Natanson C. The role of inflammation in sepsis and septic shock: a meta-analysis of both clinical and preclinical trials of anti-inflammatory therapies. In: Gallin JI SR, editor. Inflammation: Basic Principles and Correlates: Lippincott-Raven; 1999. p 965-976.
3. Root R, Dale, DC. Granulocyte colony-stimulating factor and granulocyte-macrophage colony-stimulating factor: comparisons and potential for use in the treatment of infections in nonneutropenic patients. J Infect Dis 1999;179((Suppl 2)):S342-52.
4. Nelson S, Summer WR. Innate immunity, cytokines, and pulmonary host defense. In: Infectious Disease Clinics of North America. Volume 12; 1998. p 555-567.
5. Nelson S, Belknap SM, Carlson RW, Dale D, DeBoisblanc, Farkas S, Fotheringham N, Ho H, Marrie T, Hassan M, Root R, Wilson J. A randomized controlled trial of filgrastim as an adjunct to antibiotics for treatment of hospitalized patients with community-acquired pneumonia. J Infect Dis 1998;178:1075-80.
6. Root RK. Granulocyte colony-stimulating factor in the treatment of severe pneumonia: studies in patients with sepsis and septic shock and/or multilobar pneumonia. . First International Congress on Cytokines and Chemokines in Infectious Diseases; 1999. p A134.
7. Hammond W, Csiba E, Canin A, Hockman H, Souza LM, Layton JE, Dale DC. Chronic neutropenia - a new canine model induced by human granulocyte colony-stimulating factor. J Clin Invest 1991;87(2):704-710.
8. Hammond W, Price TH, Sonta LM, Dale DC. Treatment of cyclic neutropenia with granulocyte colony-stimulating factor. N Engl J Med 1989;320:1306-11.
9. Hebert J, O'Reilly M, Gamelli RL. Protective effect of recombinant human granulocyte colony-stimulating factor against pneumococcal infections in splenectomized mice. Arch Surg 1990;125:1075-1078.
10. Mooney D, Gamelli RL, O'Reilly M, Hebert JC. Recombinant human granulocyte colony-stimulating factor and *Pseudomonas* burn wound sepsis. Arch Surg 1988;123:1353-1357.
11. O'Reilly M, Silver GM, Greenhalgh DG, Gamelli RL, Davis JH, Hebert JC. Treatment of intra-abdominal infection with granulocyte colony-stimulating factor. J Trauma 1992;33(5):679-682.

12. Nelson S, Summer W, Bagby G, Nakamura C, Stewart L, Lipscomb G, Andresen J. Granulocyte colony-stimulating factor enhances pulmonary host defenses in normal and ethanol-treated rats. J Infect Dis 1991;164:901-906.
13. Kanazawa M, Ishizaka A, Hasegawa N, Suzuki Y, Yokoyama T. Granulocyte colony-stimulating factor does not enhance endotoxin-induced acute lung injury in guinea pigs. Am Rev Resp Dis 1992;145:1030-1035.
14. Fink M, O'Sullivan BP, Menconi MJ, Wollert SP, Wang H, Youssef ME, Bellelsle JM. Effect of granulocyte colony-stimulating factor on systemic and pulmonary responses to endotoxin in pigs. J Trauma 1993;34(4):571-578.
15. Koizumi T, Kubo K, Shinozaki S, Koyama S, Kobayashi T, Sekiguchi M. Granulocyte colony-stimulating factor does not exacerbate endotoxin-induced lung injury in sheep. Am Rev Respir Dis 1993;148:132-137.
16. DeBoisblanc B, Mason CM, Andresen J, Logan E, Bear MB, Johnson S, Shellito J, Summer WR, Nelson S. Phase 1 safety trial of Filgrastim (r-metHuG-CSF) in non-neutropenic patients with severe community-acquired pneumonia. Resp Med 1997;91:387-394.
17. Hustinex W, Van Kessel CPM, Heezius E, Burgers S, Lammers JW, Hoepelman IM. Effects of granulocyte colony-stimulating factor (G-CSF) treatment on granulocyte function and receptor expression in patients with ventilator-dependent pneumonia. Clin Exp Immunol 1998;112:334-340.
18. Endo S, Inada K, Inoue Y, Yamada Y, Takakuwa T, Kasai T, Nakae H, Kuwata Y, Hoshi S, Yashida M. Evaluation of recombinant human granulocyte colony-stimulating factor (rhG-CSF) therapy in granulopoetic patients complicated with sepsis. Curr Med Res Opin 1994;13(4):233-239.
19. Gross-Weege W, Weiss M, Schneider M, Wenning M, Harms B, Dumon K, Ohmann C, Röher H.-D. Safety of a low-dosage Filgrastim (rhG-CSF) treatment in non-neutropenic surgical intensive care patients with an inflammatory process. Intensive Care Med 1997;23:16-22.
20. Ishikawa K, Tanaka H, Matsuoka T, Shimazu T, Yoshioka T, Sugimoto H. Recombinant human granulocyte colony-stimulating factor attenuates inflammatory responses in septic patients with neutropenia. J Trauma 1998;44(6):1047-1055.
21. Nishida T, Hasegawa J, Nakao K, Fujita N. Granulocyte colony-stimulating factor for gastrointestinal perforation in patients with leukopenia. J Trauma 1996;40(5):727-732.
22. Gough A, Clapperton M, Rolando N, Foster AVM, Philpott-Howard J, Edmonds ME. Randomised placebo-controlled trial of granulocyte-colony stimulating factor in diabetic foot infection. Lancet 1997;350:855-859.
23. Wunderwink R, Leeper KV, Schein RMH, Nelson S, DeBoisblanc B, Baker F, Fotheringham N, Logann E. Clinical response to figrastim in pneumonia with severe sepsis. . Am J Resp Crit Care Med; 1996;153:A123.
24. Eichacker P, Waisman Y, Natanson C, Farese A, Hoffman WD, Banks SM, MacVittie. Cardiopulmonary effects of granulocyte colony-stimulating factor in a canine model of bacterial sepsis. J Appl Physiol 1994;77(5):2366-2373.
25. Quezado Z, Natanson C, Hoffman WD, Karzai W, Koev C, Danner RL, Banks SM, Wilson L, Eichacker PQ. Granulocyte colony stimulating factor (G-CSF) treatment at the onset of *E. coli*-peritonitis-induced septic shock in canines. Am J Resp Crit Care Med 1995;151:A447.
26. Eichacker P, Hammond W, Farese A, Hoffman WD, Danner RL, Banks SM, MacVittie TJ, Natanson C. Serial serum granulocyte colony stimulating factor levels in a canine model of bacterial sepsis. Clin Res 1993;41:240.

27. Dunne J, Dunkin BJK, Nelson S, White JC. Effects of granulocyte colony stimulating factor in a nonneutropenic rodent model of *Escherichia coli* peritonitis. J Surg Res 1996;61:348-354.
28. Villa P, Shaklee CL, Meazza C, Agnello D, Ghezzi P, Senaldi G. Granulocyte colony-stimulating factor and antibiotics in the prophylaxis of a murine model of polymicrobial peritonitis and sepsis. J Infect Dis 1998;178(471-477).
29. Lorenz W, Reimund KP, Weitzel F, Celik I, Kurnatowski M, Schneider C, Mannheim W, Heiske A, Neumann K, Sitter H, Rothmund M. Granulocyte colony-stimulating factor prophylaxis before operation protects against lethal consequences of postoperative peritonitis. Surg 1997;116(5):925-934.
30. Goya T, Torisu M, Doi F, Yoshida T. Effects of granulocyte colony stimulating factor and monobactam antibiotics (Aztreonam) on neutrophil functions in sepsis. Clin Immunol Immunop 1993;69(3):278-284.
31. Smith W, Sumnicht GE, Sharpe RW, Samuelson D, Millard FE. Granulocyte colony-stimulating factor versus placebo in addition to penicillin G in a randomized blinded study of gram negative pneumonia sepsis: analysis of survival and multisystem organ failure. Blood 1995;86(4):1301-1309.
32. Frank U, Chambers HF. Treatment of *staphylococcus aureus* catheter-related infection and infective endocarditis with granulocyte colony-stimulating factor in the experimental rabbit model. Antimicrob Agents Ch 1996;40(5):1308-1310.
33. Silver G, Gamelli RL, O'Reilly M. The beneficial effect of granulocyte colony-stimulating factor (G-CSF) in combination with gentamicin on survival after *Pseudomonas* burn wound infection. Surg 1989;106:452-456.
34. Weiss M, Gross-Weege W, Schneider M, Neidhardt H, Liebert S, Mirow N, Wernet P. Enhancement of neutrophil function by *in vivo* filgrastim treatment for prophylaxis of sepsis in surgical intensive care patients. J Crit Care 1995;10(1):21-26.
35. Heard SO, Fink MP, Gamelli RL, Solomkin JS, Joshi M, Trask AL, Fabian TC, Hudson LD, Gerold KB, Logan ED. Effect of prophylactic administration of recombinant human granulocyte colony-stimulating factor (filgrastim) on the frequency of nosocomial infections in patients with acute traumatic brain injury or cerebral hemorrhage. Critical Care Medicine 1998;26(4):748-754.
36. Freeman BD, Quezado Z, Zeni F, Natanson C, Danner RL, Banks S, Quezado M, Fitz Y, Bacher J, Eichacker PQ. rG-CSF reduces endotoxemia and improves survival during *E-coli* pneumonia. Journal of Applied Physiology 1997;83(5):1467-1475.
37. Freeman BD, Correa R, Karzai W, Natanson C, Patterson M, Banks S, Fitz Y, Danner RL, Wilson L, Eichacker PQ. Controlled trials of rG-CSF and CD11b-directed MAb during hyperoxia and E-coli pneumonia in rats. J Appl Physiol 1996;80(6):2066-2076.
38. Karzai W, von Specht BU, Parent C, Haberstroh J, Wollersen K, Natanson C, Banks SM, Eichacker PQ. G-CSF during Escherichia coli versus Staphylococcus aureus pneumonia in rats has fundamentally different and opposite effects. Am J Resp Crit Care Med 1999;159(5):1377-1382.
39. Eichacker P, Quezado M, Zeni F, Correa R, Rontana J, Banks S, Fitz Y, Danner RL, Natanson C. G-CSF increases or decreases the relative risk of death dependent on site and severity of infection in rats. Am J Resp Crit Care Med 1996;153:A252.
40. Karzai W, Eichacker PQ, Mehlorn B, Bloos F, Reinhart K. The role of neutrophils in ventilation induced lung injury. Anesthesiology 1999;91:A1394.
41. Eichacker P. Prophylactic granulocyte colony-stimulating factor in critically ill patients: not time yet. Crit Care Med 1998;26(4):636-637.

INDEX

U

V

W